D1640369

DR. ROB JONES

PROTECT YOUR BACK 101

Easy Steps to Fix Your Painful Back and Prevent It From Returning

For my parents, Jon and Mary, who gave me the two greatest gifts: love and an education. For my beautiful, sweet, smart girls, Emma and Addison who show me constant love and joy in spite of their Dad sometimes being a grumpy old bugger. Most of all for my wife, Shannon, whose always there for me with honest, Zen-like wisdom, humor to always crack us up and an unbreakable, selfless love and spirit that never stops giving.

Thank you for purchasing *Protect Your Back 101.*

Please download the exercise videos and bonus content at the following link:

www.heydrrob.com/pyb101

Download QR Reader for your digital device.

https://itunes.apple.com/us/app/qr-reader-for-iphone/id368494609?mt=8

https://play.google.com/store/apps/details?id=uk.tapmedia.qrreader&hl=en

Contents

Changing the Back Pain Paradigm
So You Can Live Pain Free

Foreword

by John Novosel Jr.

If you've ever had back problems this book is for you.

If you work out, this book is for you.

So, let me re-cap: If you've had back problems and/or workout, this book is a MUST read.

Why?

Well, there is a lot of misinformation on back pain and even more misinformation on training, especially training the core. The current paradigm is that if we workout (the core), then that will protect our back... I say: 'au contraire mon frere'.

Why you ask?

Because, there are some rules the body adheres to. Rules that can't be broken. These rules are similar to gravity. There's no debate: if you throw a rock up it will come down. Nothing can stop that. When you break these rules, the body breaks down and injury and dysfunction occur. These rules aren't randomly selected. They are based on real hard science from the leading experts in the world. Here's the problem, an epidemic of improper application of exercise is being taught and practiced in the fitness industry and training world. In many cases what you are reading and what you are being taught is flat out WRONG! And it doesn't make a difference if you have a certified personal trainer helping you. Many trainers are up to date with the science but unfortunately, many are not. So, you're either working out and potentially hurting your back, or you're paying someone to hurt your back! Which leads to my story.

I've been a golfer all my life and I was into the fitness thing at an early age. I've always tried to stretch, workout, do cardio, you know all the standard stuff. And I always had lower back problems, which I could never figure out, because I was in shape and worked out. I've been in the golf business in so many different ways. I do commercials and invent training aids and work on books and teach golfers and have many certifications. I've even competed in long drive, reaching distances of over 400 yards! I worked extensively on my swing and fitness and in 2006 I started to compete with swing speeds of 135 plus miles per hour and ball speeds over 195 miles per hour. Our first child wasn't born yet, so I really poured everything into it. By the end of that year, I had herniated a disc in my lower back and had unbearable sciatic pain. I tried all the holistic ways to heal my injury, but nothing worked. I eventually had to get steroid injections. Thankfully they worked. But I was left wondering, 'is this going to happen to me again'?

Enter Dr. Rob Jones.

For my rehab, I went to see Dr. Rob Jones. He's a local chiropractor in my town. I won't lie, I was skeptical at first. How is he going to prevent this awful pain from returning? One of the first things you see with Dr. Rob is that this guy is strong! Not that that really matters, but it tells you that he practices what he preaches. He put me at ease with his knowledge of the body and his many years of clinical experience with my type of injury. He took the time to educate me on how these injuries occur and what we will do to ensure it doesn't return. He formulated a program and exercises specific to my injury and then he explained to me how to take care of my back. What was most shocking to me was the fact that he wanted me to continue working out but he had specific things that I should NOT do!

It was one of those moments when you feel like someone had punched you in the chest. I had been breaking all the rules. I was doing it all wrong and this led to all of my back problems! The even more shocking part was I was doing the exercises that the 'industry' considered the best to develop my core for performance in my chosen sport! I was doing what I thought and had been taught were all the right things. But unfortunately for me and my discs, I wasn't because the current paradigm was completely wrong!

But why did I trust Dr. Rob? How did I know that he had found the way? After a few sessions I got better, so that was huge, because to me, results are KING. But another reason was story after story that Dr. Rob told me and they went something like this: A patient walks into Dr. Rob's office and says "my lower back hurts" so Dr. Rob does the usually poking and prodding and examining, and then asks the question that has really started him down this path to understanding the body and the back: "what were you doing that caused this injury?" On many occasions, the answer he got was: "my back has been hurting as of late so I got online, went to my trainer, did yoga, did Pilates etc. because I needed to get my core stronger to fix my back". The common trend seemed to be the same for many of these back-pain patients, the wrong exercises actually causing and/or perpetuating their back problems! There are a few variables but it always boiled down to moving the lumbar spine during the workout and/or putting the lumbar spine under a heavy load with lots of repetition (like a crunch or a sit-up). And if it wasn't from exercise, the patient might tell Dr. Rob about the way they sit (too much flexion/slumping or for too long) or doing yard work, or household chores such as laundry or twisting quickly to catch a falling child. The pattern was quite obvious.

Dr. Rob showed me that I was no different than all his other back-pain sufferers, we all tended to fall into very similar categories, improper movement creating strain on the lower back. Dr. Rob got me through my injury, changed my training, my movement and the health of my body and I know he can do it for you. I have gone the past 11 years with NO back pain. Dr. Rob educated me so I know what to do and what not to do. The principles he taught me are all laid out in this book. I do Dr. Rob's exercises every day and I do most of Dr. Rob's core exercises to keep my back healthy and to ensure I'm staying in top form. What's most amazing to me is my back does NOT hurt after I play golf or after a workout or even from doing yardwork and all three used to create hours and days worth of pain for me. I owe that all to Dr. Rob Jones. You too can learn the ways of the lumbar spine and become a back Jedi Knight like me. Trust me it will change your life, it did for me and you will thank Dr. Rob for it.

PROTECT
YOUR BACK
101

Introduction

by Dr. Rob Jones

My name is Rob Jones. I am 46 years old and like you and millions of Americans I've been dealing with lower back pain for years. I started having back problems over 20 years ago as a student trying to get in shape for athletics. I followed the advice of the "experts" in magazines and in the fitness world. I worked hard and did my crunches, sit-ups and twisting movements to develop a strong core and some decent abs but unfortunately I also developed a really bad disc problem in my lower back. So, I followed the advice of my doctor and physical therapist and did even more core work to strengthen my back. What was confounding to me was every time I did my core work, my back hurt even worse! Does that story sound familiar? My injured patients tell me daily that in spite of being compliant and doing their core work, yoga and stretching they continue to have lower back pain. Have you fallen victim to the antiquated advice of lying on your back and stretching knees to chest and doing crunches and sit-ups to strengthen away the pain? Have you further irritated your back by taking the advice of a fitness expert and bent over to touch your toes to stretch the pain away? If you have, and like me it didn't work, you're reading the right book. You see, I've been a practicing chiropractor for over 18 years and in that time, I've compiled *very specific techniques on how to fix most back problems in very few steps.* In this book, I'm going to share with you how to *prevent back injury* in the first place and, if you are currently having lower back pain, how to fix *your injury,* as well as ways to *prevent it from coming back.* Have you ever asked yourself the question "Is your exercise routine hurting you?" I wish I had! Unfortunately, there were no warnings about the damage that can be sustained by the lower back discs while doing sit-ups and crunches! What you say? Sit-ups are bad for your back? I know, you've been doing sit-ups since primary school, but I'm here to tell you unequivocally yes! Sit-ups are terrible for your lower back! In fact, I call them Dr. Rob's number one "back breaker" (more on this later). Abdominal exercise staples like sit-ups, crunches, Russian twists and many others should be red flagged and jettisoned from your exercise routine. There are myriad other exercises that are at the same danger level and unfortunately, they are still commonly recommended in exercise routines, in magazines, on DVD's and online. I'm sure it's quite shocking to hear but if you are following any of these routines even if given to you by an "exercise professional", believe me when I say that it's not a matter of *IF* you are going to break down but *WHEN!*

You see the body is designed to move in a certain way, a path of ideal function if you will. When moved along said path, the body is quite efficient at performing basic tasks, handling load and repetition and thus resisting breakdown. Keeping to this path of ideal function, the body operates well, it strengthens, it hypertrophies (increases muscle size) it becomes anabolic (a positive state of growth). It can do amazing things like lift excessively heavy weights, jump high and run fast. But stray from this path (as yours truly has done oh so many times) and the load, repetition, strain and resultant damage are more than the body's restorative capabilities can withstand and the body becomes catabolic (a state of breakdown). Muscles strains, ligament sprains, disc bulges/herniations and tears become the reality of exercise programming that was supposed to build up your body not break it down. This rings especially true if you're over 40 (like me). As a more mature adult, your body has some mileage on it and its restorative capacities are certainly not what they once were. As such, the magazine headlines espousing exercise programs that will build "A Firm Butt and Sexy Core for Your Next Vacation" or "Six Pack Abs for Pool Season" are not only perilous endeavors for you and me alike but should be avoided at all costs. Why you ask? Because your body can't move that way any longer and if you attempt to force it to do exercises that aren't indicated for your skeletal maturity, the results can be catastrophic. As a clinician with over 18 years of experience, I've witnessed so many training injuries that it would be useless to count. Muscles strains and herniated discs from sit ups (Dr. Rob's Number One Back Breaker!) and crunches are just the start.

So let's stop right here and right now and learn how to exercise ***properly*** for our advancing age. This book will give you the knowledge you need for that time when a personal trainer or an exercise class instructor attempts to move your 50 year old body through an exercise that would break down a 15 year old so that you can say "No! I'm NOT doing that move! It's on Dr. Rob's Back Breaker list"! Let's move toward getting *stronger,* more <u>stable</u> (in the areas that are designed for stability—more on this later!) and flexible (in the areas that are designed for flexibility) and *fix those painful areas* that are hindering your quality of life with well-designed exercises that were screened by a clinician who applies them every day in his practice. Let's take out all the guess work and risk and instead ensure that your exercise always helps you and NEVER hurts you.

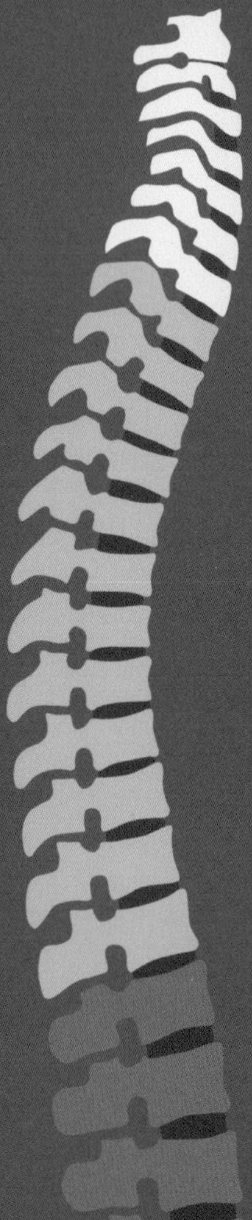

1
How The Body Works—
The Stability/Mobility Continuum

Repetitive Strain Disorder/Injury

Aside from traumatic events like auto wrecks and sprains and strains, most injuries that we sustain as mature adults fall into the category known as repetitive strain/cumulative trauma disorders. What the heck is a repetitive strain disorder you ask? Simple: it's an injury sustained simply by moving incorrectly over and over and over again. Rotator cuff impingement or tendonitis, lumbar disc bulges and tension headaches are all repetitive strain disorders. As stated previously, when the body is performing movement along its path of ideal function, or neutral position, very little strain is placed on the tendons, muscles, ligaments, nerves and joints. But stray from that neutral position just slightly and the forces of load increase exponentially resulting in strain to your muscles, tendons, ligaments and nerves. Take sitting at a computer or using a hand held device for example. Every inch of forward head movement made while looking down at your phone/device, places roughly 10-15 pounds of load (from the weight of the skull and its contents) on the musculature of the neck and upper back. Research shows that most people using a device or computer carry their heads on average 3-5 inches forward from neutral. Do the math and you'll see that's roughly 50-60 pounds of load your neck and shoulder blade musculature have to withstand! While the head is in that forward position, the muscles on the back of the neck and between the shoulder blades receive signals from the brain saying, "Hey! You're in a bad position! Contract and pull the head back to neutral!" Most of us ignore those signals until it's too late and the muscles begin to tighten and tighten and tighten. That's when pain sets in. No wonder tension headaches and upper back/neck stiffness are so pervasive. Technology is putting our bodies into positions they can't sustain without injury. A slight change of the head back to neutral performed every few minutes can correct the strain almost immediately (more on this later).

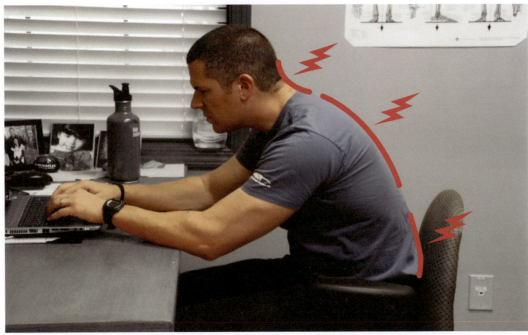

Notice as the head moves further forward the spinal curves leave their neutral/safe position creating spinal strain, muscle tightness and spasm and pain.

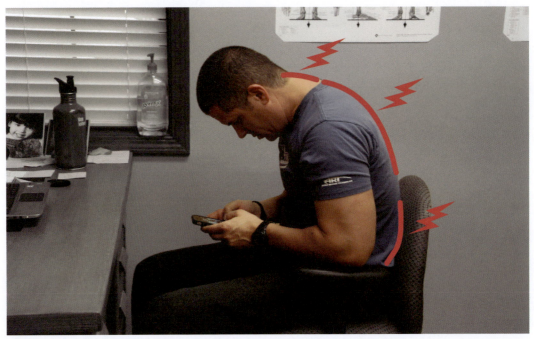

Again, note the strain to the entire spine as the neutral/safe curves are reversed.

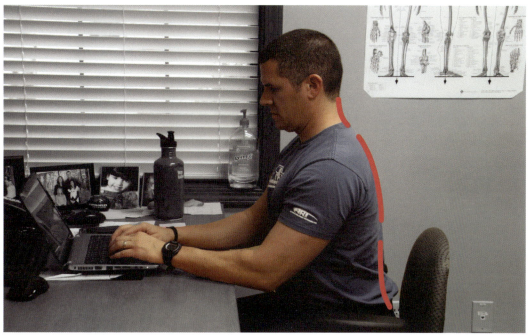

Proper sitting posture with normal spinal curves and no strain.

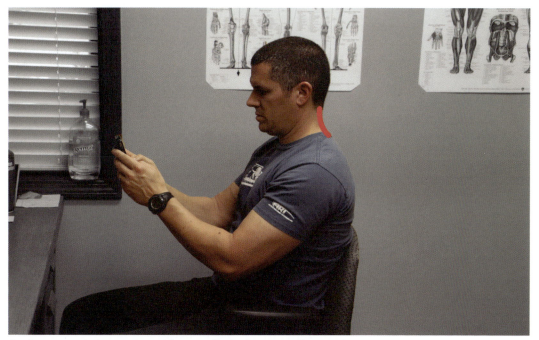

Again, proper sitting posture with normal spinal curves and no strain.

So now that you understand what a repetitive strain disorder is, let's talk about why they happen from a more global anatomical perspective. As I stated previously, the body has a tremendous capacity to do amazing things, when it's in the proper position and is following its path of ideal function. Taken off that path and it will almost immediately start to strain. Now I'm not saying you have to move like a robot and stay in position perfectly all the time: that's impossible even for a chiropractor! The body can handle small loads while out of position for short durations of time. If the load is small and the repetitions are few, then the relative risk is going to be low because the body does have the ability to repair itself when it can keep up to the insult. But if the insult is high (lots of load from weight lifting or moving your body incorrectly) and repetitive such as performing an improper exercise at the gym (a sit up) or doing yard work at home while in a position that isn't ideal, your injury risk is increased significantly without proper positioning.

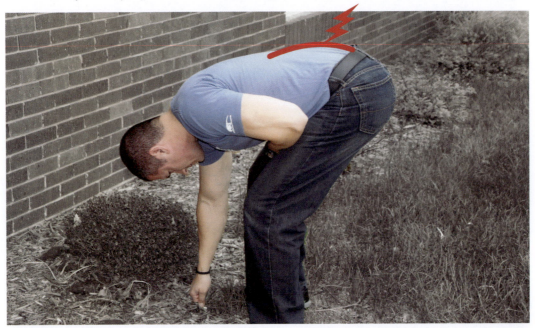

Bending forward with the low back rounded places high amounts of load and strain to the discs creating the probability of disc injury and pain.

The Spine

Let's start with the spine. For our purposes the three main areas of concern are: 1. The Cervical spine (neck), 2. The Thoracic spine (thorax/rib cage area), and 3. The Lumbar spine (low back).

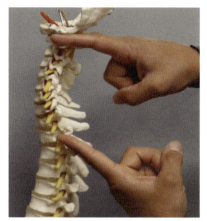

Cervical spine/neck

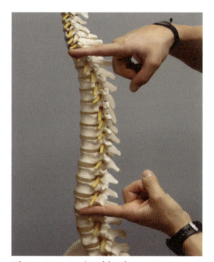

Thoracic spine/mid back

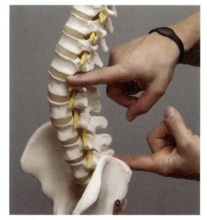

Lumbar spine/lower back

From a simple bio-mechanical perspective, all three areas must work as one to create what is called structural rigidity. Without structural rigidity, the spine isn't able to create a stable platform for the rest of the body to move from. Research has shown that if the spine isn't prioritized from a structural standpoint, exertion of strength and power through the extremities (arms and legs) is significantly minimized (more on this later). So in basic terms, it's important to remember that each area of the spine has a very specific function and, if not kept in a very specific position, that function cannot be performed efficiently leading to strain. From the bottom up, the functions are as follows: *lumbar spine (low back) = <u>STABILITY</u>, thoracic spine (mid back/thorax/rib cage) = <u>MOBILITY</u>, cervical spine (neck) = <u>STABILITY</u>.* Re-stated in the simplest terms: the more you use any of these three areas beyond their respective function the risk of breakdown is high. If you use the three areas of the spine within their stated function, then risk of breakdown is relatively low. It's as simple as that!

The Lumbar Spine (lower back)

My favorite example when explaining to patients why their low back hurts is the function of the lumbar spine (low back). It can bend forward yes; in fact, its joints are arranged to facilitate forward bending. But if forward bending is performed too often like doing sit ups (Dr. Rob's number one Back Breaker) or bending over to do toe touches in yoga, then you are creating movement in an area that craves stability NOT mobility. The lumbar spine is almost always in peril because as we age it's just easy to sit slumped, bend over to pick up our kids or grab something off of the floor. In doing so, we take the lumbar spine out of its craved c/curve (lordosis) which is its most stable position and place it into *flexion* its most *unstable* position. Usually by the age of 40, we've performed so many bends in flexion that we've gone beyond our body's ability to repair itself in that area. The ligaments that cover and protect the discs start to wear down and the results are disc bulges and herniations (more on this in the injury section). To counteract this wearing down, our exercise should *never* use *flexion* and daily movements should have a very low frequency of flexing forward from the lower back. Instead, movement forward should be through the hips (more on this in the lumbar section). To reiterate, the lumbar spine is designed for *stability:* if you don't over flex, it won't break down. Simple right?

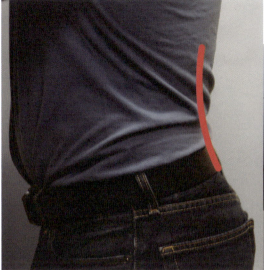

Normal/safe lumbar curve known as "lordosis".

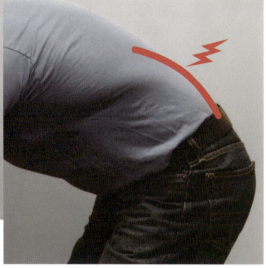

Unsafe lumbar curve with reversed lordosis; the cause of most lower back injuries.

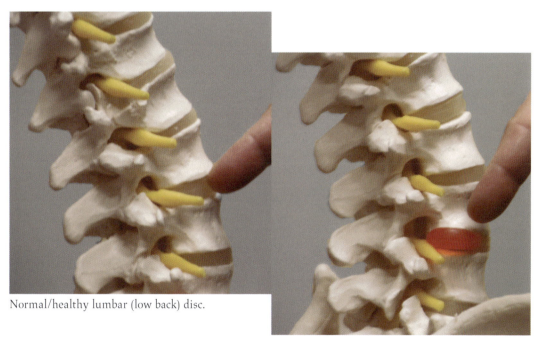

Normal/healthy lumbar (low back) disc.

Bulging (unhealthy and potentially painful) lumbar disc. Created by too much forward bending and rounding of the lumbar spine.

The Thoracic Spine (thorax/rib cage)

In opposition to the lumbar spine, the thoracic spine (mid back/thorax/rib cage area) is designed to handle a lot of movement. Its joints are set up to allow for repetitive rotation, flexing and extending (within reason of course). Let's take the golf swing for example. When the best golfers are in their takeaway, the rotation/shoulder turn happens through the movement of the thoracic spine sparing the lumbar spine from potentially straining amounts of rotation. When the thoracic spine stiffens over time due to poor posture from sitting, tightness in the chest muscles and lack of strength in the muscles that keep the thoracic spine upright occurs, the result is a loss of movement in the thoracic joints and general stiffness in the thoracic spine. I see this in clinical practice every day. An individual with a desk job sits for copious amounts of time at a desk causing the thoracic spine to stiffen which results in the lumbar spine picking up the slack for what the thoracic spine cannot do. So now we've taken an area that should be mobile and free to move (the thoracic spine), stiffened it because of lifestyle and transferred its movement to the lower back, an area that is designed to stay stable! This is why patients with low back pain often have very stiff upper backs/thoracic spines. So when treating the low back, I always address the thoracic spine to restore proper motion and spare the low back further distress from bearing the brunt of the movement. Does your lower back hurt when you swing a golf club? Perhaps your thoracic spine is too stiff and inflexible!

The Cervical Spine (neck)

The cervical spine (neck) is similar in shape to the lumbar spine, and it too craves a C/curve or lordosis. When it's in its lordosis/C-curve, the cervical spine is stable and the supportive muscles tend to stay relaxed. But when the C/curve is straightened, reversed or hyper-extended (like as it is in a typical computer posture) the muscles automatically tighten in an attempt to pull the cervical spine back into its desired lordotic position. If the cervical posture isn't corrected frequently during computer work or while exercising, its stability is lost and repetitive strain follows; tension headaches, neck pain and shoulder blade "knots" are not far off.

Hips and Shoulders

Now that we understand the proper roles of each area of the spine (movement in the thoracic region and stability in the lumbar and cervical regions), it's important to understand the role of the extremity joints (arms and legs) in relation to the spine. Without getting too bogged down in technical anatomical jargon: simply remembering what is supposed to be mobile and what is supposed to be stable is sufficient and of utmost importance. Just remember these 2 rules: 1. If you excessively move the stable joints (i. e. the lumbar and cervical regions) while performing exercise or activities of daily living, you significantly increase your risk of injury (an example is moving the lower back excessively with sits ups and toe touches). 2. If you keep the stable areas stable and move the mobile areas (i. e. the thoracic area) you significantly lower your risk for injury. It's that simple!

So, which joints are used for mobility? The ball and socket joints are your movers and shakers. If you look at them anatomically, you'll see that the ball has a smooth round surface that fits securely into sockets that also have smooth surfaces. Ball and socket joints have freedom of motion in many different directions. For the purposes of exercise and general movement the shoulder joints are your main upper body movement generators and the hip joints are your main lower body movement generators.

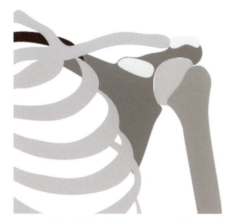

The mobile ball and socket joint of the left shoulder.

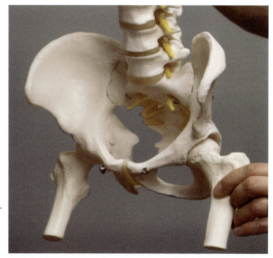

The mobile ball and socket joint of the left hip.

It's important to remember that while we can, in fact, generate movement with areas of the body that are designed for stability (again, the lumbar spine performing a sit-up for example) the movement is always less efficient, less powerful and, most importantly, it leads to breakdown. But by coupling the stability of an area like the lumbar spine and using the strongest muscles in the body (the glutes/buttock muscles) to generate movement through the ball and socket hip joints, great feats of strength and athletics can be performed. That exact sequence is how a golf ball is driven over 300 yards, how basketballs can be dunked and how power lifters can squat over 1000 pounds! Like me, your goals may not be to lift your house off of its foundation. By using the sequence of mobile joints to perform activities and stable areas to keep everything from collapsing you can effectively move through your day without causing repetitive strain, prevent injuries from occurring and most importantly move with less pain and better function. Even the simple act of standing up from a chair can be very painful if you have lower back issues. So instead of bending forward to stand up, simply keep the spine stable by raising your chest up (thus keeping the lower back in a good stable position) and use the glute muscles and hips to rise. Pain will be eliminated almost instantly. I teach chronic low back pain sufferers every day in my clinic simple tasks such as sitting down and standing up properly and you'd be amazed at the difference it can make in someone's pain and quality of life when that one simple act is changed and the strain and pain are reduced.

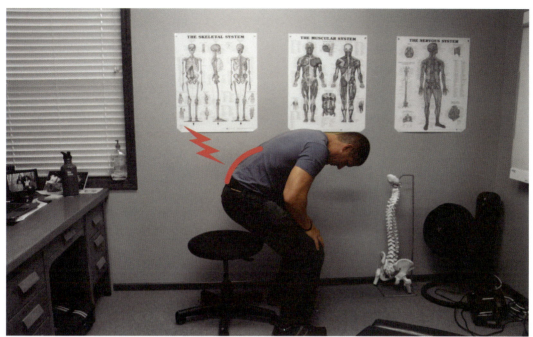

Standing incorrectly reverses the lordosis of the lumbar spine creating high amounts of load and strain on the muscles and discs potentially exacerbating current painful discs or creating new disc injury.

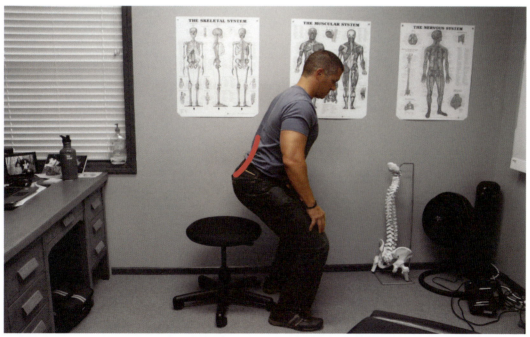

Standing from a seated position while keeping the lumbar curve in its safe lordosis creates no strain and is usually pain free for individuals with acute low back pain.

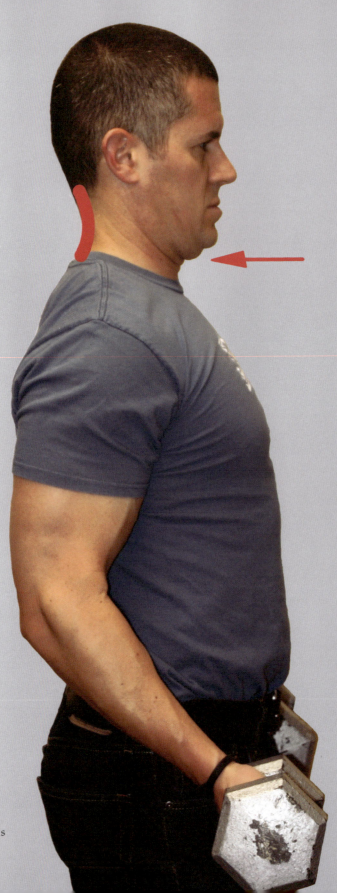

Normal cervical/neck lordosis
with neck retraction/packing.

2

What Causes Injury— How the Core Works

"The act of not moving during the presence of movement is neuromuscular stabilization (true core training)."
—*Gray Cook*

Always Prioritize Your Spine to Prevent Injury

Now that you have a basic understanding of how the spine works for stability and mobility and how the ball and socket joints of the hips and shoulders create efficient movement let's talk about how to cause an injury and how to prevent it. Simply put, if your spine is not prioritized PRIOR to any movement your system will break down almost immediately. Try this simple exercise at home: pick up an object that is relatively heavy (not too heavy please!) like a ten-pound dumbbell or its equivalent, for example. Now brace your core muscles as if someone were going to punch you (abdominal/core set/brace), pull your shoulder blades back and down to raise your chest up like a proud lion (scapular/shoulder blade setting) and pull your neck and head back like you're trying to give yourself a double chin (neck packing). Now raise that dumbbell straight forward to the level of your eyes. It should feel relatively heavy but still be manageable (If 10 pounds feels too heavy and you're straining, try less weight), now look straight up at the ceiling. Did you feel that? If you were in the proper spine prioritized position you should've felt like the weight was manageable but as soon as you looked up the weight should've felt instantly heavier and thus harder to hold up. What you were experiencing was your brain saying you are no longer in a good stable position. The neurological alarm was sounding, your brain perceived a potential injury threat and reduced the power to the shoulder muscles that were holding up the dumbbell. As a result

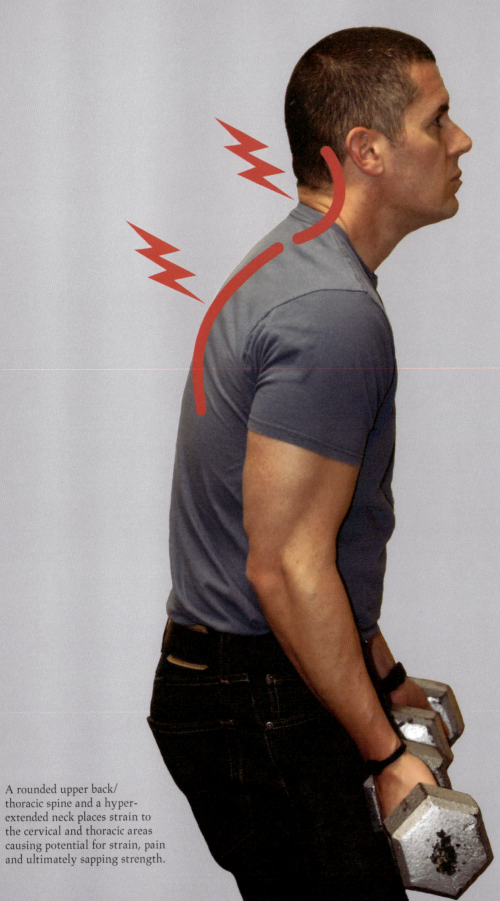

A rounded upper back/
thoracic spine and a hyper-
extended neck places strain to
the cervical and thoracic areas
causing potential for strain, pain
and ultimately sapping strength.

of this power drop the shoulder muscles (deltoids, rotator cuff and traps) had to work significantly harder to achieve a relatively menial task. Now extrapolate this to activities of daily living, your workouts or your job positioning. If you are constantly moving throughout your day without a spine prioritized position you are unknowingly creating a constant barrage of insult to your tissues! This is the exact mechanism of injury for many rotator cuff, neck/shoulder blade, tension headache and lower back injuries! I can't tell you how many times I've had patients come to me for a sore shoulder and say "Dr. Rob I don't know what I did but my shoulder is killing me!". Well now you know the answer; if you're moving through life in a poor position even the most trivial tasks can be straining!

So we've seen what can happen when the spine isn't prioritized from the top. What about the bottom? You'll need a partner for this test. Sit on a high bed or high stool and put yourself in the exact spine prioritized position we previously tested.

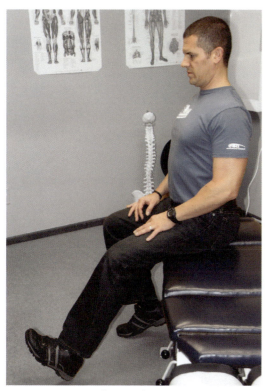

Testing position with a good strong posture. Notice how strong you are.

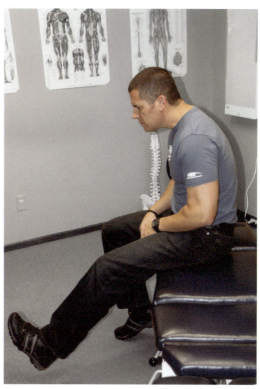

Testing position with an improper low back position/ poor posture. Notice how weak you are.

Now pull your toes upward by hinging your ankle. Have someone press down on your foot and try to resist them. What you'll notice is you were able to resist that downward force quite easily. Now slump forward so you've lost your lordosis in the lumbar spine. Have your partner apply the same amount of pressure to your foot and again resist that pressure. Did you notice what happened? It was much harder to resist, wasn't it! Again, with your spine out of its safe and stable position (this time from the lumbar area), the brain perceived a threat, sounded the injury alarms and reduced the power to your lower extremity! Imagine the amount of strain you are placing on your legs and low back while sitting in this poor position all day at your computer. Simple movements like standing up from your desk become more arduous and even something as simple as walking can be straining if your spine is not prioritized!

What is the Core?

Now that we understand the importance of prioritizing the spine prior to movement, an understanding of the stability that the core offers and how it stabilizes while the ball and sockets move the body is of utmost importance. What is the core? It seems to be all you're hearing about now in the fitness world. There are copious headlines in magazines about the core's importance and how to work it for a beautiful bikini body or six pack abs. There are many claims made that if you follow a certain core strengthening program you'll eliminate back pain. Go to any gym or fitness center and you'll find hour long classes dedicated to working the core. Unfortunately, the fitness industry hasn't kept up with the science. Aside from a few good sources, much of the core training you will see on exercise DVDs, in fitness facilities or in magazines is not just incorrect but downright dangerous for the health of your spine! When I'm doing speaking engagements and I ask the audience to tell me exercises that will strengthen the core, without fail someone will yell out "sit-ups!", then someone else will yell out "crunches!". What I'm going to say next will go against everything you have been told. Unfortunately, we've been lead to believe from early on the gold standard for core strength is the sit up. Since primary school gym class and middle school sports practice the sit-up has been used as both a source of fitness measurement and as a source of punishment. The military and some law enforcement yearly testing still require a sit up test!

So why am I picking on the poor sit-up? It's because it's THE number one Dr. Rob Back Breaker. It basically breaks all the rules of the core. The core's job is to stop movement of the spine in the presence of movement NOT create movement. I'm going to repeat that last statement because it is so important. The role of the core is *TO STOP MOVEMENT OF THE SPINE IN THE PRESENCE OF MOVEMENT <u>NOT</u> CREATE MOVEMENT!!!!* The basic nature of the sit-up places the spine in the weakened out-of-lordosis position we talked about previously. What's more, the sit-up only uses *20%* of abdominal musculature to generate the movement with the hip flexors creating the other *80%!* Not much core engagement but a great way to create disc herniations in your lower back without doing very much good for your abs!

So if the core's function is to stop motion, what exactly does that mean? Well let's look at it from a functional standpoint. If you think of the spine as a cell tower and the muscles that surround the spine as the guy wires, it's easy to understand the function of the core muscles.

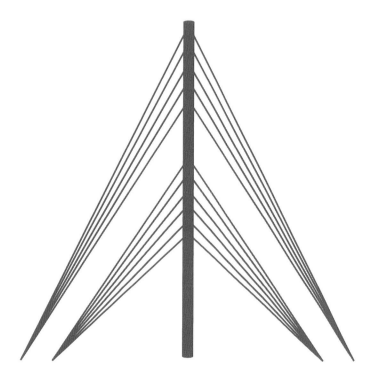

Note how the guy wires create stability for the tower. Without these guy wires the tower would be susceptible to falling over and being damaged.

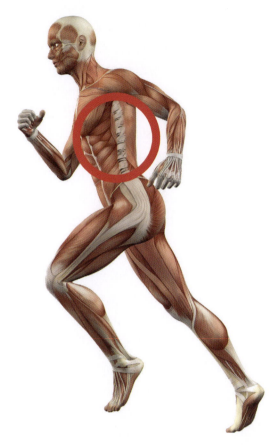

Note how the core muscles surround the spine just like the guy wires do for the tower creating stability and strength.

If the front, back and left and right sides of the torso muscles are engaged/contracting properly, the spine is stable, rigid, protected and ready to perform an activity. If one of the muscles isn't contracting properly, the spine is at risk of moving too much and thus at risk of breakdown. Think again of the cell tower: with even tension around all sides of the tower, it won't move when stressed by incredibly strong winds. But if you lose even one of those guy wires the integrity of the tower is lost and even a small amount of wind force can do damage. The spine is no different. If you keep the spine in its good stable lordotic position and engage the core to create optimal stability, new injuries can be prevented and old injuries can be ameliorated! So if you want to have a sore lower back, disc herniations and joint and muscle wear and tear, go ahead and follow your fitness instructor, your exercise DVD or your favorite magazine's "core" exercise routine and do hundreds of twisting crunches, sit ups and other spine moving core exercises. If you want to learn how to train your core properly for back safety, pain relief and overall spinal health, read on!

The Bottom Line—_The role of the core is to STOP motion of the spine NOT create motion!_

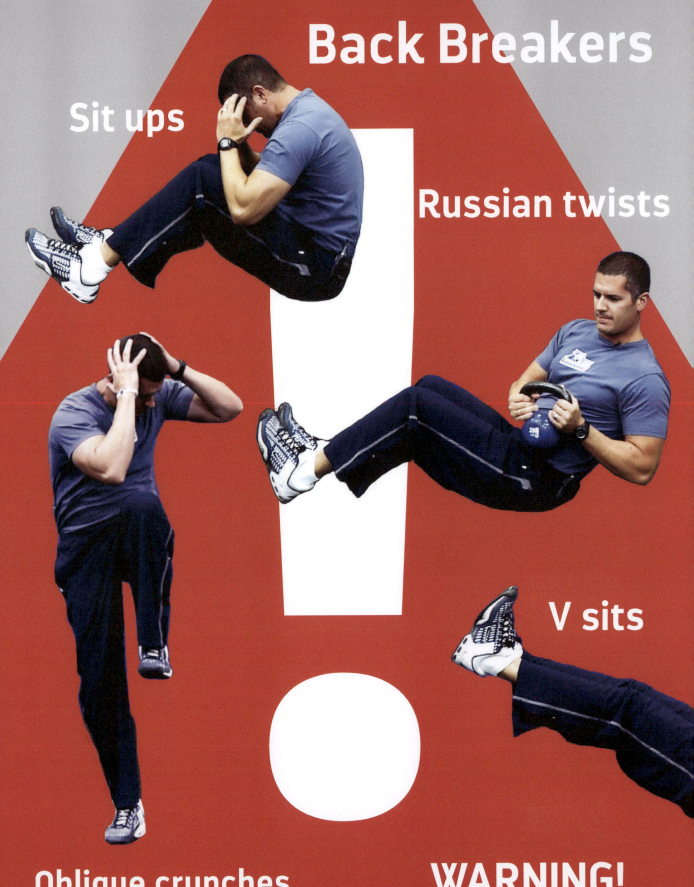

3

Easy Steps to Fix Your Sore Back

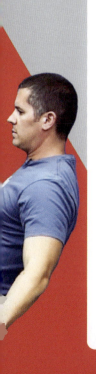

"Statistically those that have a greater range of motion in the spine have a greater risk of back disorders in the future." —Stuart McGill, PHD

The above quote from renowned lumbar spine researcher Dr. Stuart McGill is one of my favorites and one I use daily with my low back patients. Not an hour goes by in my practice that I don't treat chronic and acute low back pain sufferers that are hurt from improper movement. Unfortunately, the cause is often one's exercise regimen. As we've discussed previously there are a plethora of exercise DVDs and fitness classes that will attempt to work the core by moving the spine with what I so proudly call Dr. Rob's "Back Breakers". Please remember if you are doing any of these back breakers, it's not a matter of if but WHEN you are going to do damage to your spine and start to experience symptoms in the form of pain. Again, I can't reiterate this point enough, *if the spine is moving during exercise it is breaking down! It's that simple!* As Dr. McGill states, if you are increasing your lumbar range of motion by bending over to touch your toes, lying on your back and twisting your legs from side to side to "stretch" the low back or if you are simply lying on your back and pulling your knees to your chest (like many yoga poses), you are increasing the range of motion in your low back and creating a potential back problem. What you should be focusing on is increasing the STABILITY of your lower back with proper core work (keep reading!) and increasing the flexibility of your glutes and hips so movement can be performed through the ball and socket joints and NOT the lumbar spine.

Back Breakers

Sit-ups

Russian twists

Crunches

Bicycle crunches

Oblique crunches

V sits

V ups

Deep Squats

Toe touches

Burpees

Back Breakers

Supermans/extensions

Hyper extensions from a bench

Knee raises from hanging abdominal board

Lying knees to chest

Crunches on a ball

Side lying crunches

Side lying sit ups

Not maintaining Lordosis during a dead lift or squat

WARNING! Do not do these exercises.

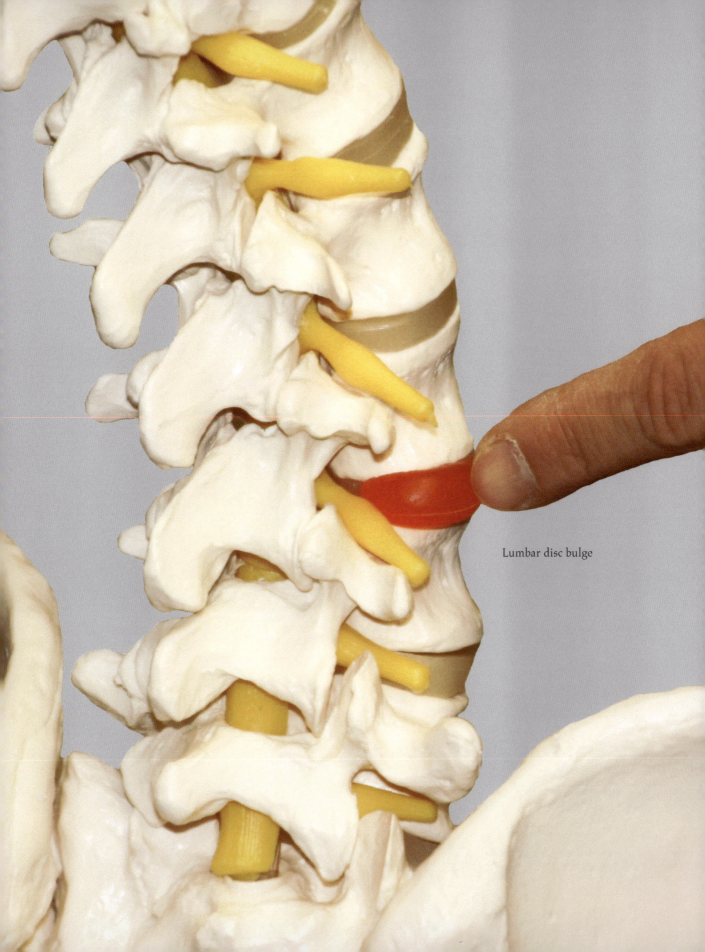

Lumbar disc bulge

4

Easy Steps to Fix a FLEXION (too much forward bending) Injury

A Great Way to Injure Your Lower Back Discs

Alright, let's work your core! Let's give you those six pack abs like your favorite Hollywood star had in his/her last blockbuster! Ready? Get on the ground, press your low back into the floor and curl up 50 times for some ab roasting sit ups! Now lock your fingers behind your head pull your knees to your chest and try to crunch away those love handles; 100 times, go! Now let's torch that fat around the mid-section by doing some burpees! Ready? 50 reps; go! Ok now that you've roasted all that fat and trained that future six pack lets cool down with some nice deep toe touch stretches to the opposite foot while we're sitting here on the ground. 10 touches per side; go! Now let's lie on our backs and stretch that lower back by rotating our legs over to the other side. You feel that lower back stretch? Good; hold it for 20 seconds and repeat four times. Does any of that sound familiar? Well if it does, it's because it's a very common "core" routine and "cool down" seen in numerous amounts of exercise DVDs or in group fitness classes. And guess what? It's one of the quickest ways to create disc bulges and really bad back pain! Yes, it might work your core slightly and get your heart rate up but it is breaking all of Dr. Rob's Back Breaker rules! Do you want to know why? That routine moved the spine with each move! Remember the lumbar spine craves stability! *If you move it during exercise you are damaging the discs, joints, nerves and muscle.* As I stated previously most of us over the age of 35-40 have flexed and moved the back thousands upon thousands of times with everyday activities, as such we absolutely cannot move it during exercise! Again, spine movement during exercise equals injury! If you can only remember and take away one thing from this entire section, it's my last point—*movement of the lumbar spine during exercise injures the discs and creates back pain!!!!!*

Understanding Flexion and How it Hurts Your Lower Back

So now you know some great moves on how to injure your discs, break the spine down and cause injury and pain. How about learning some great moves to make your core really strong, help your back pain and prevent it from coming back! First, I'd like you to understand the elements of what breaks down during what we call a *flexion cycle*. *A __flexion cycle__ simply stated is the act of taking the lower back through a range of motion in which it bends forward.* When the lumbar spine is neutral in its lordosis it forms a nice C-curve. During a forward bend or flexion cycle, it reverses that C-curve and loses lordosis. In doing so it loses its ability to stabilize itself placing all the load and strain directly on the discs.

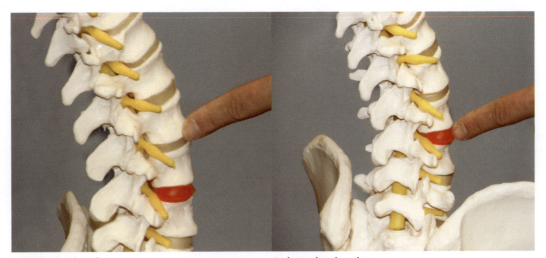

Healthy lumbar disc   Bulging lumbar disc

Too many of these flexion cycles over time with activities of daily living or with copious amounts of crunches and sit-ups place excessive strain on the back of the discs. The lumbar discs are like jelly donuts: overstress them and a structure called the annulus fibrosis (the donut portion of the disc) starts to weaken and break down. As a result, the nucleus pulposis (the jelly portion of the disc) won't be held in place by the annulus fibrosis (donut) and the "jelly" will start to leak out. As a result, bulging occurs, followed by herniation, extrusion and fragmenting. All are technical ways of saying your back is going to REALLY hurt and possibly even cause pain to shoot into your buttock and down your leg (sciatica).

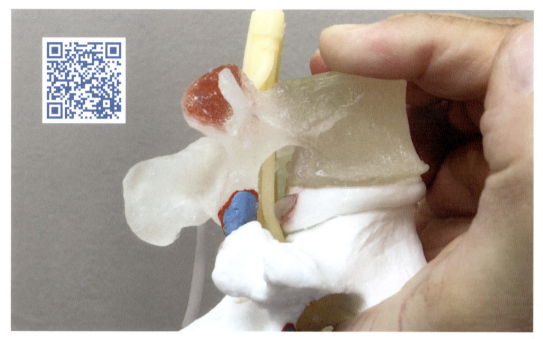

Bulging lumbar disc - Note on this disc model how when the front of the disc is compressed (like flexing/bending forward) the disc bulges backward toward the spinal cord and the nerves. This occurs over time with repeated bending from flexing with activities of daily living or with exercises such as crunches and sit ups. The more the spine is flexed, the further the disc bulges back increasing lower back pain and sciatica.

There are times while performing the activities of daily living when flexing our spines seems unavoidable (sitting, bending forward to wash our faces etc.). I typically advise my patients with back problems to completely eliminate these movements (flexion cycles) while they actively have a bulge or herniation and are in significant pain. This can be accomplished by doing a hip hinge bend instead of a lumbar flexion cycle to bend forward (more on this later). So, knowing that we place our spines under some risk during daily movements and too much flexing can and will break the spine down causing disc bulges why are we flexing during exercise? It's because the exercise instructor/program simply doesn't understand how the back and core work. Unfortunately, not all genres of the fitness industry have kept up with the best science demonstrating the mechanisms I just spoke of for back injury. Some individuals in the fitness world have kept up with the science but unfortunately as a whole the fitness industry is lagging behind; so it's really up to you to ensure you have the knowledge and understanding of how the back works to truly protect yourself from potentially harmful exercise. (See the previous chapter on "Back Breakers" for a full list of the potentially harmful exercises.)

Symptoms of a Flexion Intolerant/Disc Injury

So now you understand what not to do but you're still in pain or you simply want to learn how to train your core without injuring your spine. Great! Let's get started. Most (not all) individuals who are suffering from *flexion intolerance* (the first steps of flexion based pain prior to a disc bulge occurring), *disc bulging, disc herniations* and general *discogenic pain* (pain originating from the discs) will have very similar symptoms. Movements throughout the day that place load or strain on the lower back discs will most likely be painful and/or feel very stiff. *Positions that either place load on the discs or take the lumbar spine out of its lordosis (neutral C-curve) such as sitting, transitioning from sitting to standing or standing to sitting, rolling over in bed, bending over to pick up objects off the ground, getting in and out of a car, sneezing or coughing, doing yard work/gardening, dressing oneself such as putting on socks and pants (I can always tell immediately that a patient has a disc injury if he or she arrives at my office for evaluation with no socks on!) and morning stiffness in the low back that makes an individual feel as though they are "85 years old"* are all signs of disc related flexion pain. Flexion/disc pain can be on one or both sides of your lower back, in the middle of your lower back, in one or both of the buttocks and can even travel down the back or front of your leg as far as your toes. Flexion/disc pain can be sharp and stabbing on flexion or with coughing/sneezing or rolling over in bed. It can be a deep aching pain while sitting and driving. Although these are not all of the symptoms of flexion/disc related pain they tend to be the most common. If any of these symptoms sound familiar, you most likely have one of the types of flexion intolerant disc injuries. As such, you must remove the act of flexing the lower back in order for your lumbar discs to heal; period! Regardless of what you see in a magazine or online or what a friend in a yoga class tells you, **stretching the low back will only irritate the problem!** The injury, as I mentioned previously, is caused by flexing the lower back. So why would you flex it to fix the problem? It makes no sense! Yes, you are stretching the muscles when you touch your toes or try to round the back to "stretch away the pain", but in doing so you are putting load on the discs and the stabilizing muscles, the spinal erectors. Muscle physiology states that you cannot stretch a loaded or contracted muscle. What that means is if you bend over to attempt a back stretch, the lumbar muscles are activating/contracting (while they are being lengthened) to try and pull you upright, so you are NOT stretching them. You are just making them tighter! This "stretching" of the back muscles is simply placing further load on the low back and thus irritating the problem! As such, you will simply intensify the tightness you are experiencing in your lower back. What the spine craves at this point is its restorative lordosis, a position where the discs no longer protrude and the muscles actually have a chance to relax.

Fixing Your Own Flexion/Disc Injury

The first move for someone with a flexion intolerant lower back problem should always be to restore lordosis. This is accomplished using a position called *Prone Lumbar Elbows.*

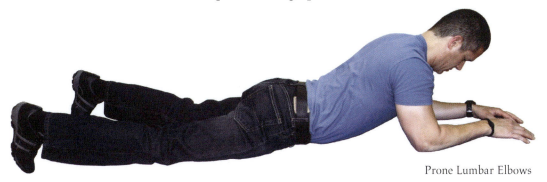

Prone Lumbar Elbows

What this move does is it starts to draw the bulging discs back into their original position by gently introducing extension. If initially the pain is too intense while on your elbows you can start with *Prone Lumbar Chin Stack.*

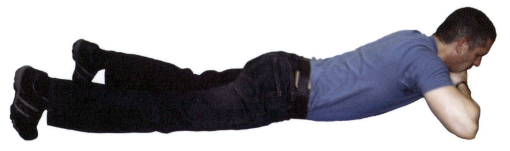

Prone Lumbar Chin Stack

As the pain begins to ease after 2-3 minutes you can change your position and carefully raise up to your elbows. After 2-3 minutes of *Prone Lumbar Elbows* a greater range of motion in extension is needed to further reduce the discs back to their non-bulging position. This second position is *Prone Lumbar Extension Presses.*

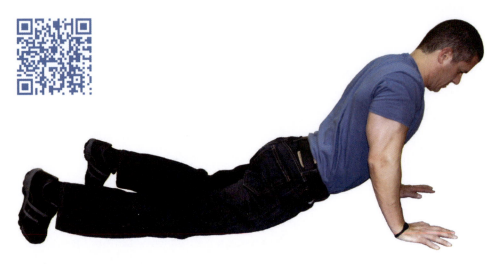

Prone Lumbar Extension Presses

This move places direct pressure on the lumbar discs and milks the bulge back into its correct position. Anywhere from 10-30 repetitions may be needed to fully force the discs back into their home. Both of these moves send the brain messages of safety, not strain, disarming the brain's danger responses of spasm and tightness. Spasms in the adjacent muscles will also start to relax. As will nerve pain down the leg as the disc lifts off of the nerve (in the case of sciatica) and the localized sharpness in the lower back (the actual pain source) will start to resolve. Two to three rounds of these floor exercises may be needed for the pain to reduce enough for you to proceed to the next exercises. What I tell my patients is to listen to what your back is telling you: if you've done one round of the prone floor exercises and the pain is still quite intense or not down to a low level such as 1-2/10 then another round or two should be attempted. Once the leg pain is moved to the low back and the low back pain is anywhere from 0-2/10 then it's time to proceed on to the next moves. Repeating the above three moves may be necessary every hour while in an acute episode of lower back pain. Once the pain is significantly diminished you can reduce the frequency of the prone moves. I usually tell my patients to do the moves more often if in pain and less often if not in pain. It's generally that simple.

Strengthening Your Core For a Flexion/Disc Injury

Now that we've started to push that angry bulged disc back into its home we need to strengthen the core musculature around the area to ensure continued stability during the activities of daily living. To start this phase your pain should be down to a low level and no longer sharp. If your pain is still sharp you should continue with Prone Lumbar Chin Stack and Elbows and Prone Lumbar Extension Presses, until your movement is more normal and your pain is significantly lowered. If the injured area is not stabilized through proper core exercises, the chance of a disc injury recurrence is high.

The first move I recommend to begin the stabilization phase of low back repair is the *Bird Dog.*

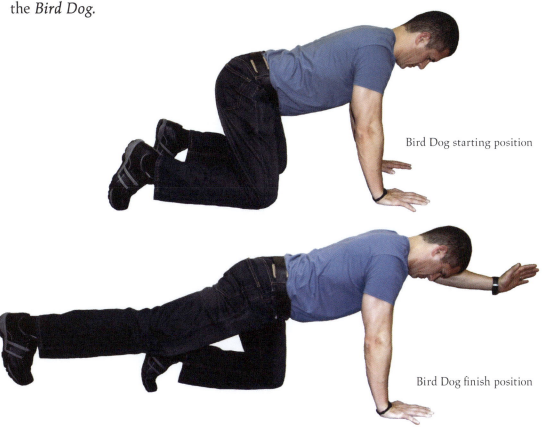

Bird Dog starting position

Bird Dog finish position

The Bird Dog is one of the best core/spine stabilizers simply because it creates good core contraction and deep muscular stimulation with very minimal load on the lumbar discs. It activates the deep core stabilizers, the rectus abdominus (abs), obliques and quadratus lumborum (the side core musculature) as well as the superficial spinal stabilizers the spinal erectors (the big muscles on either side of the spine).

The second move I recommend to my patients to restore core activation and strength is the *Dying Bug.*

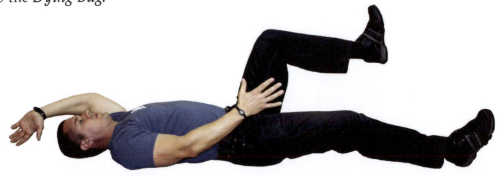

Basic Dying Bug. Core is braced (NOT pressing low back to ground), keeping lumbar lordosis arms and legs are alternating as in walking. Tap heel to the ground as you reach overhead, return to start position and repeat on the opposite side. Go until fatigued and always keep perfect form.

Much like the Bird Dog, it creates core activation to the deep and superficial stabilizing muscles of the lower back and pelvis. Another unique property of the Dying Bug is it places the lumbar spine into a nice lordosis which forces the discs back into their normal, pain-free resting place. This will help tremendously with pain as well as properly activate those very important core muscles.

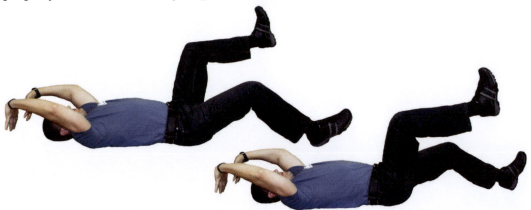

More advanced Dying Bug—the Wall Bug. While pressing vigorously against a wall keep your lumbar lordosis and tap alternating heels to the ground at a steady pace until fatigued. Again perfect form is necessary.

The third move I recommend for dealing with flexion based/disc issues and retraining the core is the *Bear.*

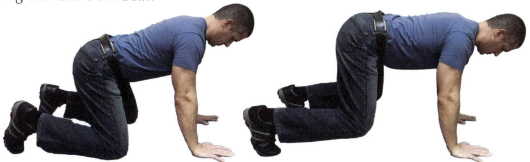

Start position for the Bear.   Hold position for the Bear.

Much like the Bird Dog and the Dying Bug it places the spine in a nice neutral position wherein the lordosis forces the discs back into position. With the mechanical load from the lordosis as well as a strong core contraction relief can be felt almost immediately when a patient with an irritated disc is placed in the Bear. With the Bear, deep and superficial core muscles work together to stabilize the spine.

Both the Bird Dog, Dying Bug, and the Bear accomplish two very important things: 1. They place the lumbar spine in a neutral, disc sparing position. 2. They create automatic core activation. The act of automating a proper core response (i.e. automatically bracing your core to protect your spine in the presence of a potentially injurious situation) is paramount to maintaining a healthy lumbar spine. Unfortunately, there is a lot of misinformation out there regarding core activation and ways to accomplish proper activation to protect your back. Many fitness instructors and physical therapists will advise individuals to draw the navel to the spine to activate the core. According to Dr. Stuart McGill, this is simply a myth, and doesn't in fact, activate enough of the core musculature. What it actually does is *destabilize* the spine. Another cue incorrectly given to patients and individuals is to press the low back into the floor while lying on their backs during exercise/rehab. Again, this is ineffective and actually injurious because it takes the spine out of lordosis (the safe position) and actually loads the discs! On the other hand, the Bird Dog and Dying Bug exercises are so effective precisely because they place the spine in a neutral lordosis and automatically contract all of the core musculature. The key to these moves is to ensure that your lordosis is where it needs to be to find the greatest amount of relief.

The Bird Dog

For the Bird Dog, assume a quadruped (all 4's position) and allow your lower back to fall comfortably toward the floor. A gentle curve/lordosis should be where you end up. If it is truly a neutral position for you, the pain should be resolved.

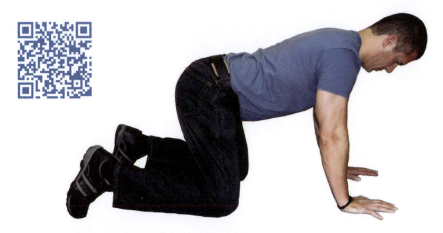

Bird Dog start position with a pain free neutral/lordotic lower back.

If the pain persists, adjust the level of lordosis by slowly moving your spine up and down until you find a comfortable position. If you still cannot achieve a pain free position, you should return to your stomach and resume Prone Lumbar Elbows and Prone Lumbar Extension Presses. Once you are out of pain then attempt the Bird Dog once again. Once you have found your lumbar neutral position, gently brace your core as though you are about to be punched. Do this by picturing an inner tube around your waste and pressing the musculature of your mid-section *outward* to fill the space between your belly, sides and lower back and the inner surface of the tube.

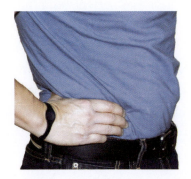

Brace the core by pressing your muscles outward as if protecting yourself from a punch. DO NOT SUCK YOUR BELLY BUTTON IN!!

Now with your head neutral and looking down at the ground raise your left arm and your right leg until they are both in line with your body.

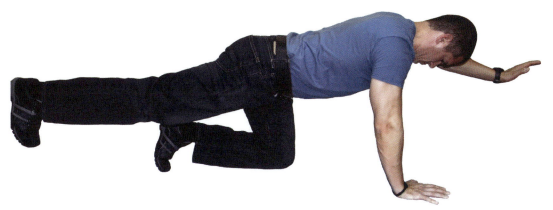

Hold position for the Bird Dog. Remember to brace your core through the entirety of each rep

Do not over elevate your leg or arm as this will create too much motion in the spine. The spine should remain stable and immobile while the ball and socket joints of the shoulders and hips create the motion. Hold this position for 3-5 seconds and return to the starting position. Now repeat on the opposite side.

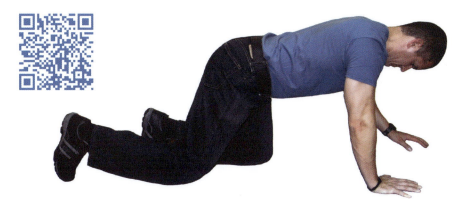

Immediately return the same arm and leg back out. The cadence for this should be 3 seconds out, hold for 3-5 seconds and 3 seconds down while maintaining a neutral lower back curve and bracing the core. Bird Dog With Sweeps. Once the basic Bird Dog is easier and your pain is reduced, after holding the arm and leg in full reach return them to the starting position by sweeping the hand and knee against the ground. Don't set them down and rest, immediately take them back out to the elevated position and repeat.

Your goal should be to do 10 repetitions per side with a 3-5 second hold per repetition. Once you can do this without straining add some repeats on each side. This is accomplished by doing a 3-5 second hold repetition and sweeping the ground at your start position and then immediately returning to the extended position.

Your goal is to do 10 sweeping repetitions with a 10 second hold on each side. Once you can perform the recommended repetitions, you will know that you are on the road to achieving a strong and protective core. I tell all my back pain patients that, as long as their lower back pain is present at low levels, these exercises should be performed daily. As your pain subsides, you can decrease the frequency of the exercises. Keep in mind, however, that as you start to feel better, you will naturally want to do more work around the house and participate in your favorite activities again which will add some additional risk to your healing back. So be sure to make the Bird Dog a part of your weekly routine so your core is continuing to strengthen on an ongoing basis and has the capacity to handle the strain of everyday living and an active lifestyle. Doing 2 sets of 10 reps with 10 second holds of the Bird Dog 3-4 times per week (coupled of course with spine sparing movements) once you are out of pain is a great way to stave off future back problems.

The Dying Bug

To do the Dying Bug lie on your back and raise your legs up to just below 90 degrees. As your legs come up to the 90/90 position your back should naturally fall into a pain-free neutral position. Do NOT attempt to press your low back to the floor!

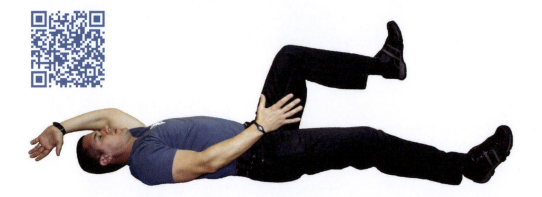

As with the Bird Dog, your spine position should be pain free. If it is not simply move your lordosis up and down slightly and you should be able to find a comfortable, pain free position. Now, moving from the hip only and NOT the knee, slowly lower one leg and tap the ground with your heel. Once you return that leg back to its starting position lower the other leg and return it to the starting position. What you'll notice about the Dying Bug is your spine will automatically move into lordosis and your core will contract as your leg is moved away from your body. If the position of your lower back is uncomfortable, simply play with your lumbar positioning until it is in its most comfortable spot. Once your lower back is comfortable, in a safe lordotic position, proceed with the exercises until you're somewhat fatigued. Rest and repeat three times. As the exercise proceeds your pain should remain low (if not gone) and a burning/fatigued feeling will be felt in your abs, low back muscles and hip flexors. This is all normal and an important step to ensuring stability in your injured lower back. By pressing your hands against a wall you are forcing your core to work very hard (yet safely!) to stabilize the spine. As you get stronger, try pressing really hard into the wall like you are holding it up. You will feel an immediate, very strong core contraction.

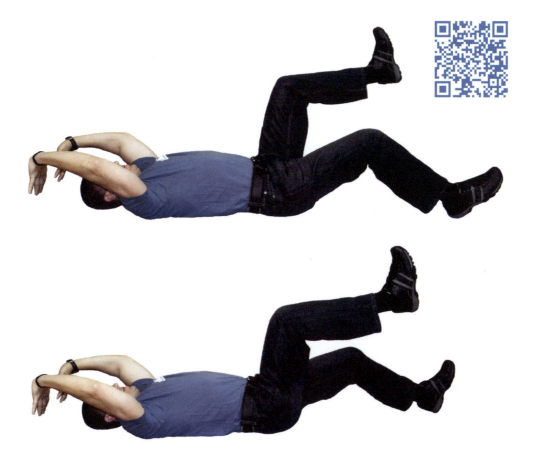

This is an automatic and responsive core contraction that is paramount to a strong, functionally stable core. As with the Bird Dog, the Dying Bug should be performed daily until you are out of pain. Once you are out of pain, performing the Dying Bug 3-4 times per week for 2-3 sets until fatigued is a great way to stay strong through your core and help prevent that back problem from returning.

The Bear

To perform the Bear, start on your hands and knees with your knees under your hips and your hands under your shoulders. You should slowly move your lumbar spine up and down until you feel a comfortable lordosis that is pain free.

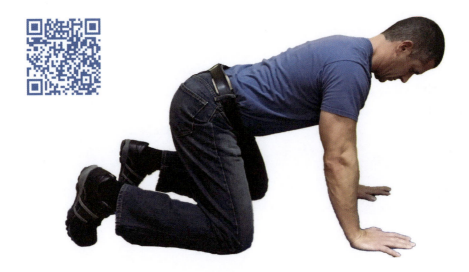

Once in that position brace your core (just like the Bird Dog and Dying Bug) and raise both knees simultaneously off the ground so your knees are roughly 4-5 inches off of the ground. Once your knees are 4-5 inches off of the ground push your knees out to the sides (away from midline) slightly (only 2-3 inches) until you feel your glutes (buttock muscles) engage. Once in this position hold for 5 seconds.

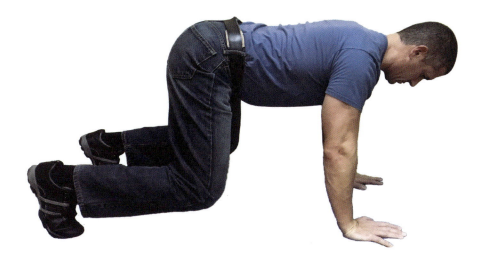

After 5 seconds lower yourself to the ground without letting go of your core. Once you are on the ground release your core, rest for 1-2 seconds and repeat. Be certain to not let your lumbar spine lordosis change as you raise up! It should remain in the same position throughout the entirety of the motion. Also, ensure you don't release your core until you are back on the ground. You should start with 5-6 reps holding each rep for 5-6 seconds. Try to do 2-3 sets of 5-6 reps daily until you feel stronger. As this becomes easier and your core strengthens you should attempt to do 7 reps holding for 7 seconds and so on until you can accomplish 2-3 sets of 10 repetitions of 10 second reps. As with the Bird Dog and Dying Bug, the Bear should be performed daily until you are out of pain. Once you are out of pain performing the Bear 3-4 times per week for 2-3 sets of 10 reps of 10 second holds is a great way to build and maintain a strong core and help prevent future back problems and relapses.

**Quick Review: Strengthen the Core to Fix Your Disc/Flexion Back Pain with the:**
1. **Bird Dog**
2. **Dying bug**
3. **Bear**

Staying Pain Free—Moving the "SOS" Way

So now you are mostly out of pain; the pain referring into your buttocks and leg is lessened, your lower back pain is not as intense while you are sitting and driving your car. Great! Now how do we keep it from coming back? This, my fellow lumbar pain sufferers, is a very important question. You see research shows that one of the greatest causes of having low back pain is being a previous low back pain sufferer. Well that stinks right! Yes, it does, but if you follow my plan you *CAN* and *WILL* prevent future low back pain episodes. As I stated previously, we know that with a flexion based injury you've simply bent over too many times. So the solution to not re-aggravating your lower back is simply to no longer flex your spine. By taking that move completely out of your repertoire we will virtually eliminate the cause of the pain! Learning how to spare your spine through hip hinging, instead of bending forward with your lumbar spine, will ensure minimal load to your back and place movement through the ball and socket joints of the hips. Moves like the forward hip bend, golfer's pick up and lunge bend need to become the new normal! If you take away the act of forward bending/lumbar flexion there will be no chronic irritation to your spine and thus no injury.

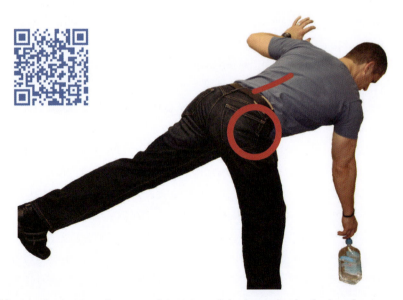

Golfer's pick up. Note the neutral position of the lower back, the hand support on the wall and the leg kicking back. The lumbar spine/low back stays neutral while all of the motion occurs through the ball and socket joint of the hips.

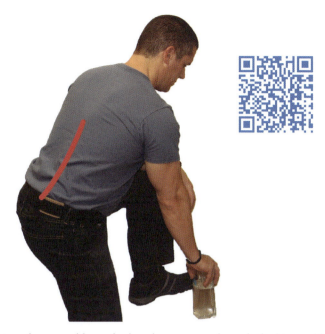

The Lunge pick up. Note the neutral lower back and movement through the hips and knees only.

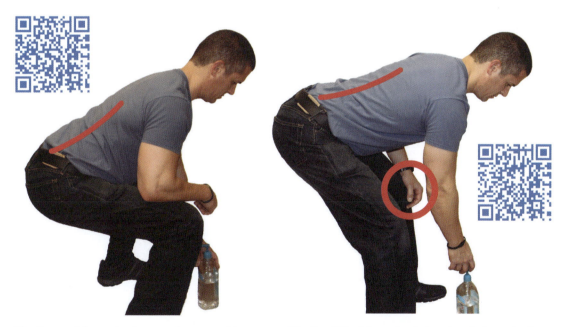

The Squat pick up. Again note the neutral lower back, support of the upper body weight on the R knee and all the movement being created through the hips and the knees NOT the lower back. If knees are painful during this move simply push your knees further away from each other (sideways).

The Deadlift pick up. Again keeping the lower back neutral movement is created through the hips. Feel for a big stretch in the hamstrings NOT the lower back; this sensation will remind you you're bending properly.

It's that simple! I teach these techniques every day in my clinic to chronic low back pain sufferers and the results are astounding. When you can actually feel the stretch in your hamstrings from a proper hip hinge bend and not in your lumbar spine from an improper lumbar bend you've taken away the insult and given your back a chance to finally start healing. It's not going to be easy: re-educating your brain and muscles to move differently never is. You've been moving in a set pattern for years and in some cases decades. You are going to have to think in a new way about your movement. So there is going to have to be a lot of effort involved. If you simply slow down and take a second or two to plan your movement, the new movement patterns will become easier, more common and eventually automatic. You can start this process by utilizing a system I call *"SOS"*: *"S"* is Stop, *"O"* is Observe/Assess what the task is, *"S"* is Start the task. By practicing this simple acronym (it only takes a second or two) you can lay out a plan of action for tasks that potentially may be injurious, and begin to create a foundation of proper movement that the motor centers in your brain can recall automatically for future tasks thus eliminating the patterning of improper movements.

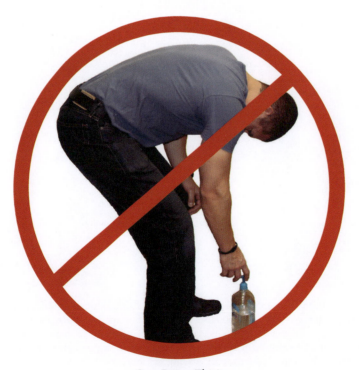

Stop Doing This!

Sitting—What a Pain in the Back and Butt!

One of the many contributing factors to lumbar flexion injury is the simple act of sitting. When we sit we put tremendous load on the lumbar discs. In fact, sitting with poor posture places the lumbar C curve in a reversed position.

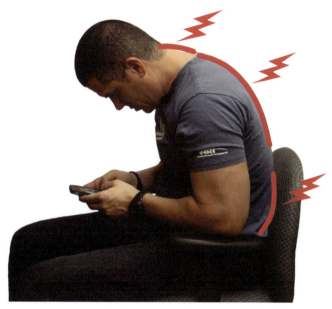

If you are in back pain or not, this position should always be avoided.

This reversed curve position, creates one of the highest amounts of straining load to the lumbar discs. So just like your mother told you so many years ago, sit up straight! Well, easier said than done right! I know first-hand how hard it is to maintain a good lumbar curve while sitting. It's very tiring to sit perfectly postural for many hours at your computer, at a ball game, on your couch etc. The two easiest ways to mitigate the strain to the discs from a poor sitting posture are: 1. Place a support behind your back and 2. Simply stand up every 15-20 minutes and do some simple back extensions. When sitting on a couch or office chair I recommend and personally use a small pillow to fill the space between the lumbar curve and the back of the chair or couch.

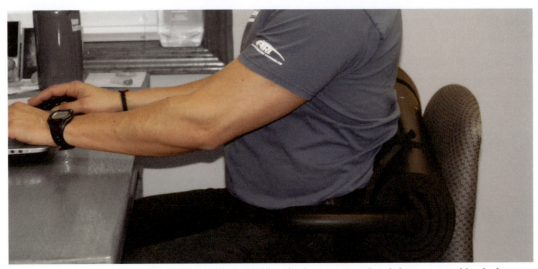

By using a pillow or other supports the lumbar spine/low back is supported and the strain and load of sitting is significantly diminished.

This props the spine up in its lordosis and supports it even if you fatigue and attempt to reverse the curve into its injurious/slumped position. If the lumbar support isn't enough to help with the pain or you are seated on bleachers (at a football game or other event) that won't allow for support then simply stand up every 15-20 minutes and do 10-20 standing back bends.

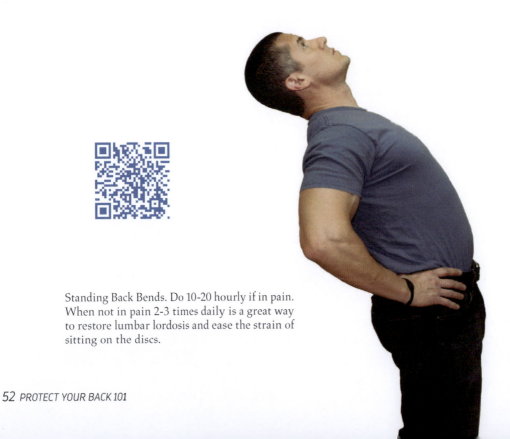

Standing Back Bends. Do 10-20 hourly if in pain. When not in pain 2-3 times daily is a great way to restore lumbar lordosis and ease the strain of sitting on the discs.

This will almost immediately reverse the curve in your low back into the safe lordotic position it craves, tuck the discs back in to their pain free position and significantly diminish your pain and stiffness. Another great way to stop the pain while sitting at work, on the couch, at a game or while driving is to do what I call Seated Extensions. Seated Extensions are very similar to standing back bends but you can remain seated. Simply sit up nice and tall with your back in lordosis, grab your knees (or the bottom of your steering wheel if you're driving) and pull toward your body. As you are pulling, arch your back as far as you can and hold for a 1 count.

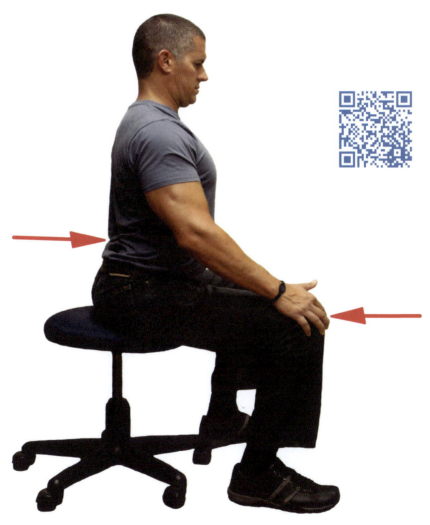

Seated Extensions. If you're in a situation that won't allow you to stand, then 10-20 reps hourly is a great way to calm low back pain. When not in pain 2-3 times per day will restore lower back lordosis while sitting and ease pressure and load on the discs.

Repeat this as many times as needed until the pain in your buttock, leg, or low back subsides. My patients typically find that 10-20 reps of Seated Extensions will ease their pain. This technique can be utilized every 15-20 minutes while sitting as long as symptoms persist. With these three easy steps sitting should no longer pose the problem it once did for your lower back pain.

> *Quick Review: To Stop Disc/Flexion Pain While Sitting:*
> *1. Place a support behind you back*
> *2. Do 15-20 Standing Extensions frequently*
> *3. Do 10-20 Seated Extensions frequently*

Ice Away Your Pain

Lower back pain is typically an inflammatory condition. What this means is your body is attempting to heal the area with inflammation. Small amounts of controlled inflammation are a good thing: it's how we heal. Too much inflammation will create longer lasting and more intense pain. This is where ice comes in handy, it's a great inflammation reducer. What I typically recommend is a regimen of 20 minutes of icing to the lumbar spine while one is lying supine (on your back, face up) 4-5 times per day after doing extension exercises, during the initial acute phase of low back pain. Once pain intensity and frequency are improving I typically recommend decreasing the frequency of icing to 1-2 times per day. Icing for 20 minutes while lying in bed just prior to sleep (be sure to not fall asleep with an ice pack on your back) is a great way to decrease inflammation prior to sleep and help you get through the night with less pain. Please stay away from heat. Many people will reach for heat because as the commercials say "heat to melt away the pain". Although the heat might feel good at the moment, low back inflammation pain will only worsen with heat. Think of it this way: heat is short term gain for long term pain and ice is short term pain for long term gain. Along with my exercise routines, icing can be an effective way to help eliminate your lower back pain.

Safe Stretching for a Flexion/Disc Injury

When my lumbar disc/flexion injury patients are out of pain they often ask me when they can start stretching again. Many are concerned their backs will stiffen without stretching. I usually have to revisit the lumbar safety talk and I can't stress enough to my patients that even when they are out of pain, the spine is very susceptible to injury if you start flexing it again. The recommendation I typically give is to stretch the glutes (buttock muscles) and psoas (hip flexors). As we've discussed previously, the hips need to be mobile and loose while the lumbar spine stays stable so glute and psoas flexibility is paramount to a healthy lumbar spine. Again, without flexible glutes and psoas the hips cannot move properly and thus forces the lumbar spine to move excessively, leading to injury. I typically teach the glute stretches sitting because they're very practical stretches; they can easily be performed while sitting at your desk or while having dinner with your family.

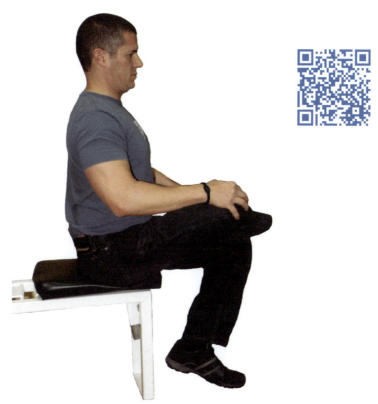

Seated Figure 4 Glute Stretch. A great practical way to stretch tight glutes while sitting. Simply cross one leg over the other, raise the down side leg heel off the ground and lean slightly forward until a glute stretch is felt. Remember DO NOT round forward; keep your back in lordosis! Hold 20-30 seconds.

Psoas stretching is also easily achieved simply by standing, spreading your legs front to back in a wide lunge stance, leaning forward and squeezing the glutes of the back leg (be sure not to extend the spine). Holding each stretch for 20-30 seconds will accomplish flexibility in both the glutes and psoas and allow for proper ranges of motion in the hips to allow for spine sparing movements and future back health.

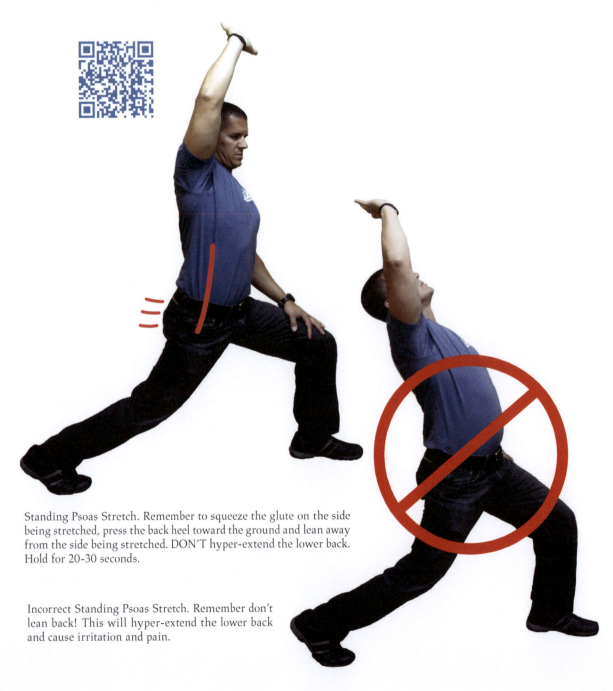

Standing Psoas Stretch. Remember to squeeze the glute on the side being stretched, press the back heel toward the ground and lean away from the side being stretched. DON'T hyper-extend the lower back. Hold for 20-30 seconds.

Incorrect Standing Psoas Stretch. Remember don't lean back! This will hyper-extend the lower back and cause irritation and pain.

Patients with healing low back injuries often feel quite stiff in the lumbar area and are typically anxious to start stretching the lower back. I recommend *NEVER* stretching the lumbar spine under load (such as bending over to touch your toes (a Dr. Rob Back Breaker).

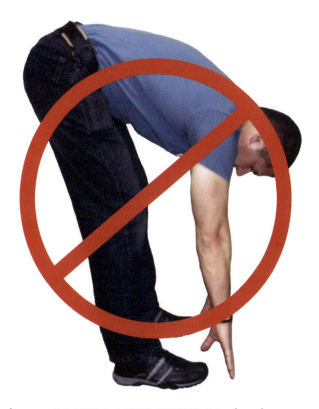

If you are in pain/injured or not, DO NOT DO THIS STRETCH! Look at the position of the lower back, rounded and susceptible to injury!

However, as long as there is *no pain* in the lower back during the activity and the spine is under *no load* the cat/camel exercise is quite effective. The Cat/Camel accomplishes three important things for the lower back: 1. It loosens stiff muscles that may have become inflexible due to injury to the area. 2. It creates proper articulation (joint range of motion) in spinal joints. 3. It flosses the nerves through the foramen (holes) where the nerves exit the spine to reach the lower extremities. The importance of creating a symbiotic balance between stability and flexibility is one of the keys to maintaining a pain free back, so utilizing the stretches for the glutes and psoas as well as the Cat/Camel are paramount to keeping you moving properly and out of pain.

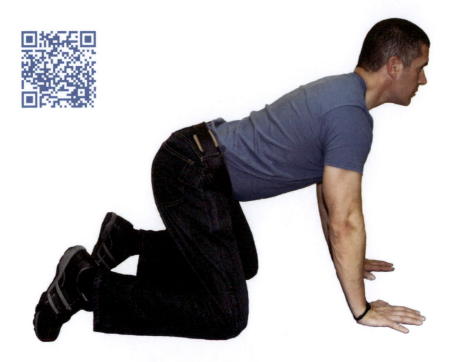

Cat/Camel Stretch. Some stiffness and mild pain that occurs at the top and the bottom of this movement is o.k. if it resolves in 5-8 repetitions. It's safe for the lower back to work through that stiffness and mild pain but if the pain persists past the 5-8 repetitions don't go as far into the range of motion that hurts as it may irritate your discs. Only work the pain free range of motion. I typically recommend 15-20 repetitions of the Cat/Camel.

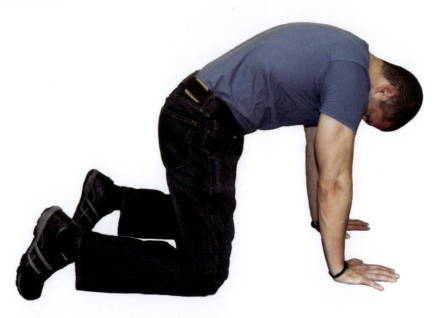

Pain Pain Stay Away!

Alright, you're out of lumbar flexion pain; fantastic! Does this mean that you can immediately clean the garage, do several hours of yard work and maybe even hit the gym for some squats and deadlifts? My patients often ask me if they can jump back in to such activities. Well, the answer is yes, and no. You can definitely start to perform your normal activities but please remember that the greatest cause of back problems is a previous back problem. So a gradual introduction of activity is indicated. Starting slowly and seeing how your body responds is of the utmost importance. Being mindful of spine sparing activities of daily living such as using a hip hinge to bend forward, using a golfer's pickup or lunge pickup will keep your back healthy and pain free. I always explain to my patients that lumbar flexion will occur in everyday life and the potentials for irritation of a lumbar disc problem are everywhere so incorporating strategically placed *prone lumbar elbows* and *prone lumbar extension presses* are extremely important to maintaining a healthy back. Even if you feel you've moved very well during several hours of yard work or during a hard exercise session, be sure to immediately follow whatever activity may have placed you at risk with 2-3 sets of *prone lumbar elbows* and *prone lumbar extension presses.* As maintenance for a healthy back this can be done daily or every other day. My patients typically find a rhythm for what works for them and they often note that the extension work will prevent most recurrences of flexion intolerant or disc based injuries. My advice to you is, find the rhythm that works for you and stick to it! A pain free lower back *IS* possible!

Toe Touching is Overrated!

Before we move on to the next type of back pain I'd like to address a question/scenario I see every day in my practice. When I see patients with low back pain in my office, especially the ones who are staunch yoga followers, they are almost always very proud of their ability to touch the floor with their hands. They will often state "I don't get it Dr. Rob! I've been able to touch my toes for years yet my back still hurts!". This is a phenomenon that we've all been dealing with for decades (for those of you that are younger maybe just years). We're taught in gym class in primary school to touch our toes is somehow a measure of fitness. During my exercise physiology labs in University we even had a "sit and reach test". Somewhere, sometime, someone determined that if you can touch your toes you must be healthy and fit. I'm here to tell you that couldn't be further from the truth! In 18 years of practice, I've only had 5 patients (yes only 5!) who could maintain their lordosis while they touched their toes or the ground. Typically, what occurs is that the individual begins to reach for the ground and as they approximate their knees their hamstrings will reach their limit of elastic range (flexibility limit). At this point the individual will slowly start to unwind their lordosis (placing it at risk) and touch their toes or the ground and in doing so micro-damaging their spine and discs. As Dr. Stuart McGill states "Those with the highest ranges of flexibility in their spines have the highest rates of injury". So what in the world are we doing touching our toes! It's a cultural phenomenon that HAS to stop! If you want to stretch your hamstrings it's quite simple, aim for your knees or your shins and call it good. Keep your spine in lordosis and only reach to the point where you cannot go any further and you feel a big hamstring stretch. That's it, no more, no less. You've accomplished a nice healthy hamstring stretch and spared your spine. Culturally what we should be seeing as a measure of health and fitness is whether or not an individual at a young age can control their spinal lordosis by keeping it stable while they flex at the hips to accomplish a hamstring stretch. By making this one small change, especially at a young age, we could potentially mitigate millions of cases of future low back injury and pain and save billions of dollars in healthcare costs.

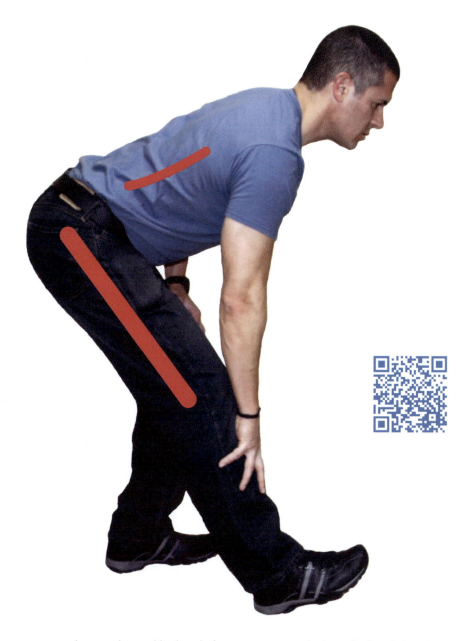

Proper Hamstring Stretch. Note the good lordosis/safe curve to protect the lower back. While in this spinal position push the hips back until you feel a big stretch in the hamstrings (back of the upper legs/thighs). There is no need to touch your toes! Reach down toward the knee until a good deep stretch is felt in your hamstrings. Touching your toes is not a good measure of health and fitness so don't worry if you can only stretch to your knee or mid shin.

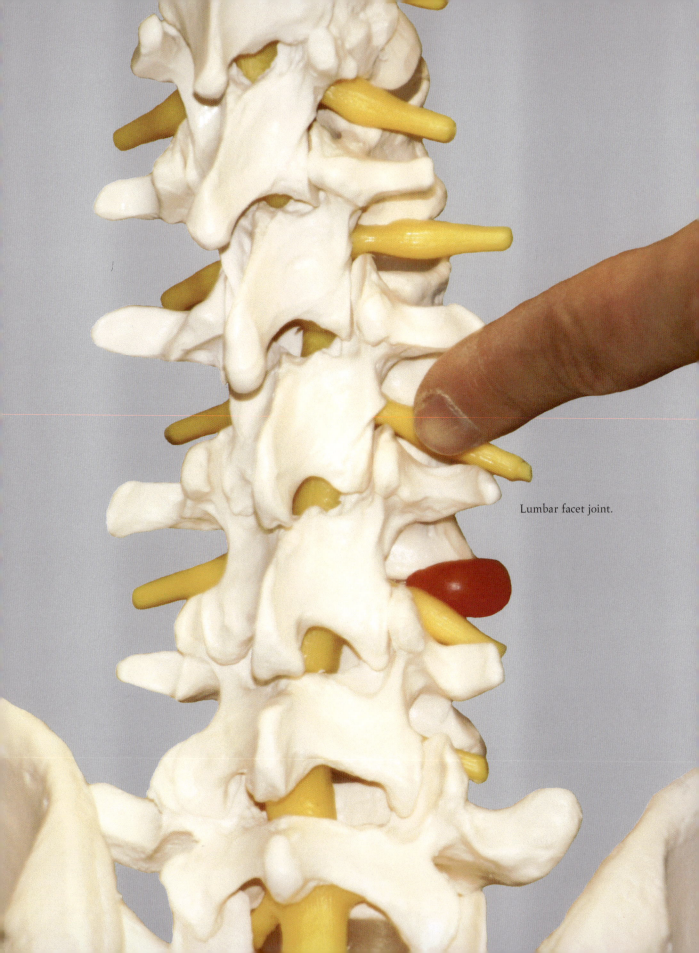

Lumbar facet joint.

5

Easy Steps to Fix an EXTENSION (too much backward bending) Injury

Extension Intolerant Back Injury

Another type of back injury I've seen over the years is the extension based injury. Although this is much less common than the previously discussed flexion based injury it can be just as painful and debilitating. Unlike flexion injuries that will break down the discs with forward bending, extension injuries do damage in exactly the opposite way. Excessive extension (backward bending) of the lumbar spine will cause facet joint and nerve issues in the lower back. In a clinical setting I typically see extension intolerant (backward bending pain) patients that fit into two categories: 1. Younger individuals that have performed excessive amounts of backward bending/extension from dancing and other athletics such as gymnastics, diving, yoga and several other sports that consistently create extension of the spine over and over and over again

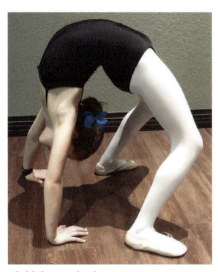
Child doing a bridge.

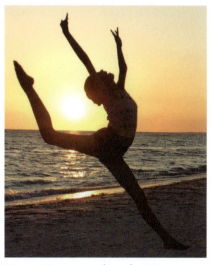
Dancer Hyperextending the Spine

and 2. Older individuals that have arthritis of the joints of the spine and stenosis (narrowing of the foramen/holes where the nerves exit the spine).

Symptoms of an Extension Intolerant Back Injury

In both cases of extension intolerant low back injuries, _pain is present and can be quite intense while bending backwards even with small ranges of extension._

What may be slightly confusing to patients is flexion intolerant/disc patients often have pain with extension as well as with their main movement pain, flexion. A quick way to differentiate if you have a flexion based injury or an extension based injury is to try some extensions. With flexion based injuries repeated extensions either on your stomach (prone lumbar extension presses) or standing, will improve extension pain after several repetitions. Extension based pain will WORSEN with repeated extension.

Both may result in localized low back pain in the center, on the right or on the left or refer pain into the buttocks and down the legs while extending the spine. Stenosis (the more serious of the two) is typically painful while standing and walking with pain referring so intensely down the buttock and leg that the individual will have to sit down or bend forward to relieve the pain even after a short walk. As with many medical conditions, there are always exceptions to the rules. Typically, the easiest way to differentiate if you are having sciatic pain from a disc issue or stenosis is your age (stenosis is usually seen in the golden years). More commonly though, _pain in the low back, buttock or leg that worsens with prolonged sitting, driving, bending forward and transitioning from a chair but is IMPROVED WITH WALKING, is typically a disc related/flexion based injury._ If sciatic (buttock, thigh and leg) pain _WORSENS WITH WALKING and one has to sit down or bend forward to alleviate the pain, stenosis or an extension based sciatica is usually suspected._ As with flexion intolerant/disc based pain, extension injured patients should learn to move properly to spare the spine. Hinging through the hips while keeping the spine in a neutral posture to take pressure off of the discs AND the facet joints and nerves is of paramount importance. Once proper movement is taught and we've eliminated the mechanism of pain for the athletic individual or the non-athletic individual we can start our rehab protocols to help the problem and ease the pain. Facet (joint) based pain can be eliminated with proper adherence to lifestyle/movement changes but stenosis is a harder nut to crack and in some cases may require referral.

Hip Extension VS. Back Extension—The Key to Fixing Your Extension Injury

What I find clinically with patients that are extension intolerant is they typically default into lumbar extension (sway back) during most exercise positions. Teaching my patients hip extension with a lumbar neutral position, is paramount to fixing this problem. I typically teach simple standing hip extension versus lumbar extension so patients can feel the difference between the two movements. Once they recognize the injurious movement (lumbar extension), they can eliminate it from daily activity and incorporate hip extension solely as that form of movement. Try this, while holding on to the wall, simply extend one leg back. If you feel pain or a compression sensation you are extending your lumbar spine and creating injury. The movement that needs to be taught and perfected is the simple hip extension while the lumbar spine stays neutral and immobilized with a core brace.

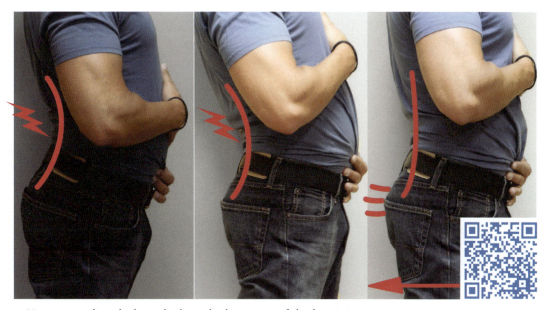

1. Hyper-extending the lower back can lead to injury of the facet joints.
2. Extending the hip and spine create hyper-extension which can irritate the facet joints causing pain.
3. Note the neutral lumbar spine/lower back stays still while THE HIP moves backward into extension thus sparing the low back.

To accomplish this, stand facing a wall or counter, hold on with both hands and brace your core to prevent the spine from moving, now slowly extend one leg back and STOP as soon as you feel your glute muscle contract. Did you feel that? That's a perfect spine sparing hip extension. If you feel pain or compression in your lower back, stop and try the movement again until you ONLY feel the glute. Once proper hip extension is accomplished and you can cognitively correct this movement fault and actually feel the glute extending the leg while the lumbar spine stays neutral, we can proceed with the rehab exercises.

The Bird Dog

With patients that are extension intolerant, I typically start their rehab with the *Bird Dog.* This move should be utilized exactly as per the previous section on flexion intolerant/disc pain suffers. As with disc injured patients the goal of the bird dog for extension intolerant patients is to teach lumbar neutral. So start in a quadruped position and drop your spine as low as it will go WITHOUT pain, now bring it up slightly so you have a safe lumbar lordosis without hyper extending your spine and without pain. This is your lumbar neutral position.

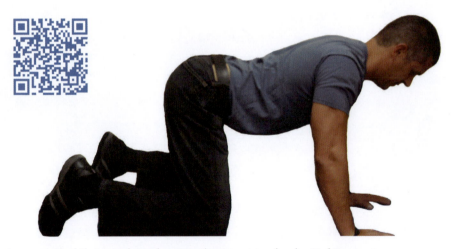

Lumbar neutral while in quadruped position/start position for the Bird Dog.

Now that you've found lumbar neutral, brace your core and lock your spine in position. Now proceed as above with the Bird Dog exercise and work up to 10 reps per side with 10 seconds of hold on each rep.

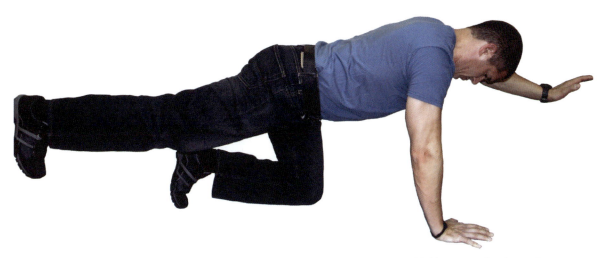

Hold Position for the Bird Dog.

The Glute Bridge

My second go to exercise for lumbar extension intolerance is the *Glute Bridge.* The Glute Bridge is a very important exercise simply because it teaches patients with extension pain to utilize the most powerful muscles in the body (the glutes) to perform the movement without defaulting to spine extension to create the movement (as during the standing extension test). Simply lie on your back and just like the Bird Dog, find a comfortable neutral spine position (slightly lordotic with no pain). Please I beg of you *DON'T PRESS YOUR LOWER BACK TO THE GROUND!!!* Although this technique has been disproven in the science and will harm your back, it is still being taught in many fitness clubs and yoga studios! It is flat out wrong and should never be used, even if one has a healthy lower back. Ok, now that I'm done with that rant let's proceed. From that neutral spine position (pain free with a slight lordotic arch) brace your core, push your knees apart and lift your hips off of the ground using your glutes and maintaining your neutral spine position throughout the entire movement. Hold this position for 3 seconds at the top, then lower your body back to the floor maintaining your neutral lumbar position.

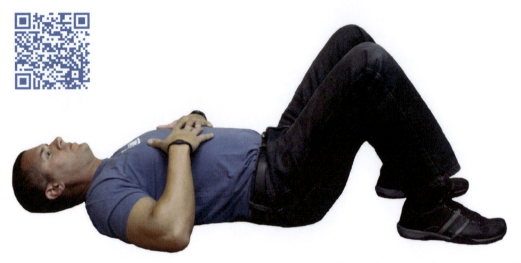

Glute Bridge with neutral spine. Movement occurs through the HIPS from a glute (buttock) contraction and NOT through the lower back/lumbar spine.

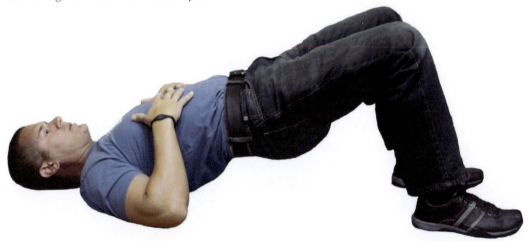

If you feel pain, then reset your lumbar position and try again. Typically, if pain is present, you are using your lower back muscles to perform the movement instead of your glutes. In many cases the glutes will simply be shut off neurologically from lack of use and over-utilization of the lumbar muscles (a very typically default pattern). If this is occurring, then simply reset your lumbar spine and start the move exactly in the same manner but only push your feet to the ground to feel your glutes engage. Don't lift your body off of the ground. Simply hold this position for 3-5 seconds and relax, reset and repeat 10-12 times. Once you can feel your glutes contracting and the lower back is no longer hurting, raise your hips off the ground so your quads (front of the thighs) are in line with your abdominals.

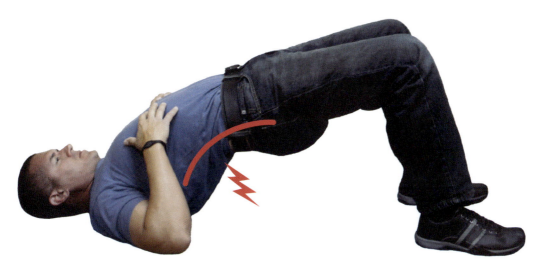

Glute Bridge with a hyper-extended lower back. Note the excessive lower back lordosis/curve placing compressive load and strain to the joints (facets) of the lower back. This movement is often painful for patients with extension intolerance. Once a neutral low back is restored at the start of the movement and glute contraction initiates the upward movement pain is usually resolved.

Be careful not to hyper-extend your spine at the top of the move. This is a very common mistake and will only irritate your lower back pain. At the top of the move a nice strong glute contraction should be felt and held for 3-5 seconds. Lower your body to the floor and reset your position and repeat the move as many times as you can until you feel fatigued. The goal should be 12-15 reps with a 2-3 second hold on each rep. When you've completed this move you should feel a nice level of fatigue in your glutes (maybe even a burn) and your pain should not be exacerbated: in fact, it should be improved. I recommend doing 2-3 sets of the glute bridge with 30 seconds break between sets on a daily basis until your pain is resolved. After pain resolution, the glute bridge is an important move to ensure your glutes continue to fire (contract) with daily use, thus sparing your low back. I typically recommend the glute bridge be performed 3-4 times per week as maintenance and as part of a healthy core program.

The ½ Side Bridge

The third exercise I utilize for extension intolerant/pain patients is the *½ Side Bridge.* Much like the Bird Dog and the Glute Bridge the ½ Side Bridge is utilized to create a nice strong, glute utilized hip extension while keeping the lumbar spine in a neutral position. Start by lying on your right or left side and propping yourself up on your elbow with your knees and hips in the 90/90 position.

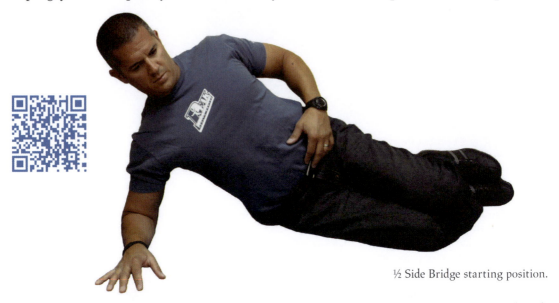

½ Side Bridge starting position.

Now, set your shoulder blades back so your chest is raised up and your shoulder is stabilized (this is called shoulder packing or centration and is actually good for rotator cuff and neck/upper back issues). Once the shoulder is set/packed draw your chin back to stabilize your neck. Now raise your lower back up toward the ceiling, so it is not sagging down to the ground, find your lumbar neutral (as you did with the Bird Dog and Glute Bridge) and brace your core.

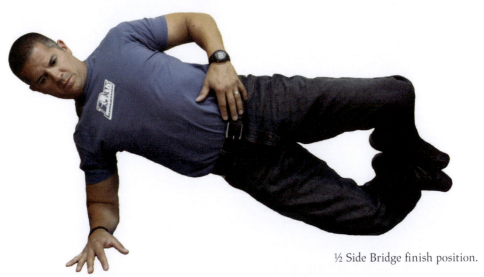

½ Side Bridge finish position.

Holding this position, drive your down side knee into the ground and push your hips forward. Just like a regular Glute Bridge you are moving your hips through a range of motion WITHOUT moving your spine. Hold at the top for 3-5 seconds and move through your hips (what we call a hip hinge) back to the start position all while maintaining that neutral spine and abdominal brace.

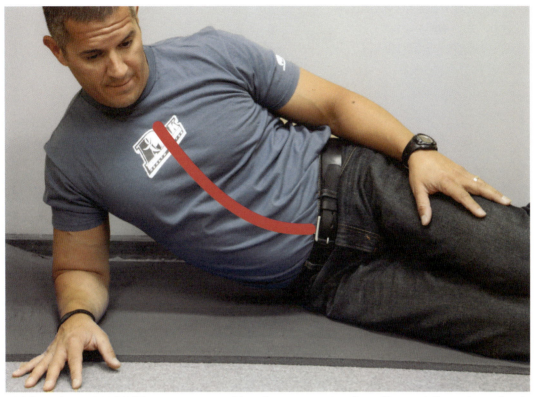

½ Side Bridge INCORRECT starting position. Note the sagging spine that will potentially strain an already painful lower back and potentially irritate a non-injured lower back.

Repeat that same movement 3-5 reps per side for 3-5 seconds each rep. Your goal on this move should be 10 reps for 10 seconds each. If there is any level of pain you're probably not starting with a neutral spine. Start over and reset your lumbar neutral and abdominal brace and proceed. You'll know that you've achieved lumbar neutral and a hip hinge/glute movement when you can do this move with no pain. In many cases of extension intolerance/pain the muscles lock the lower back into the extension posture. The psoas (hip flexors), quadratus lumborum (QLs) and glutes become tight, short and immobile. By moving through the hips, while maintaining a neutral spine, individuals can usually loosen these locked-down muscles and find relief from their pain quite quickly. If muscle tension isn't relieved by the previous three exercises stretching can be incorporated to help alleviate the pain.

__Quick Review: To Fix Extension Intolerant Low Back Injuries and Pain use:__
1. The Bird Dog
2. The Glute Bridge
3. The ½ Side Bridge

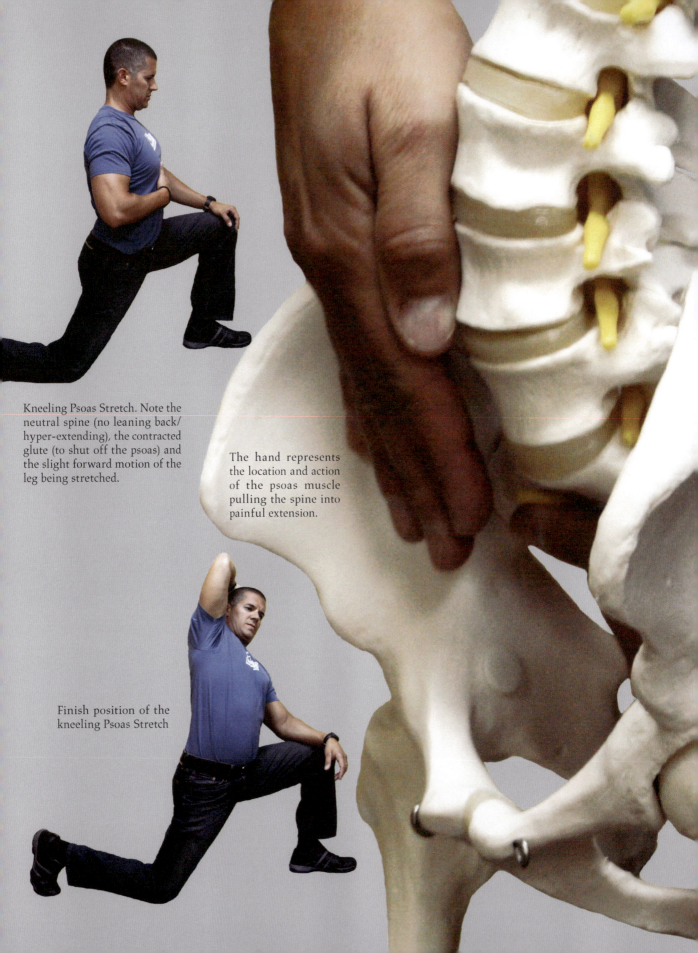

Kneeling Psoas Stretch. Note the neutral spine (no leaning back/hyper-extending), the contracted glute (to shut off the psoas) and the slight forward motion of the leg being stretched.

The hand represents the location and action of the psoas muscle pulling the spine into painful extension.

Finish position of the kneeling Psoas Stretch

6

Proper Stretching to Alleviate Extension Intolerant Back Injuries

Psoas Stretching

The psoas muscles are powerful hip flexors but when they become hypertonic (tight and short), they will draw the spine into extension and place pressure on the nerves and joints. The psoas can be stretched one of two ways. 1. Kneeling on one knee in a deep lunge position with your hips forward WITHOUT EXTENDING THE SPINE. An immediate stretch will be felt on the back leg psoas/hip flexor. By squeezing the back leg glute and leaning away from the side being stretched you will feel a really effective psoas stretch.

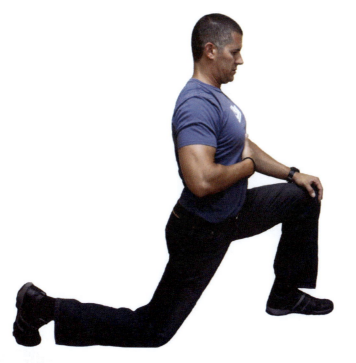

Kneeling Psoas Stretch

If you can't kneel due to a knee problem the psoas stretch can be accomplished while standing (as previously taught in the Flexion Intolerant/disc pain stretching section). Stand close to a counter or window ledge and split your stance as wide as is comfortable. Now rock your hips forward while squeezing the back leg glute.

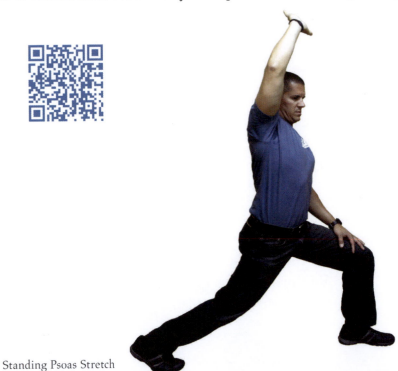

Standing Psoas Stretch

Lean away from the side being stretched and hold from 20-30 seconds. A nice deep stretch should be felt from the hip flexor (front of the back hip) all the way to the front of the abdominal wall (this sensation is the upper aspect of the psoas being stretched way up into the lumbar spine). If you feel pain in the lower back then you are extending the spine, stop and reset your position, and concentrate on squeezing the back leg glute much harder. Once you feel as though you've really got a good feel for this stretch, applying it 3-4 times per day and holding it 20-30 seconds while in pain is appropriate. When you are pain free the psoas stretch is a great stretch to keep in your repertoire for daily maintenance stretching. The psoas will tend to get tight and short with prolonged sitting (we all do too much of this!) as well as after walking, running or athletics so after activity or after long periods of sitting, 2 sets of 20-30 seconds of psoas stretching is a great way to keep your back and hips healthy and happy.

Quadratus Lumborum (QL) Stretching

When the QL muscles are tight and short, they create a compressive extension on the lumbar spine so stretching them out safely is of utmost importance. The trick to stretching the QL is not to flex the lumbar spine. Doing so will just tighten up the QLs even more. The best way to stretch the QL is to get in a ½ side lying position propped up on your hand. With your right side down, slowly press your right side toward the ground and slightly turn your left shoulder to the right. You should feel an immediate stretch in your right side.

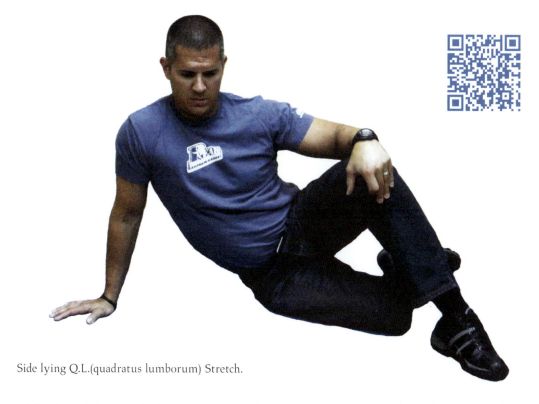

Side lying Q.L.(quadratus lumborum) Stretch.

Hold this QL stretch for 20-30 seconds 2-3 times and switch to the other side and repeat. If pain is present, you are probably pressing too hard to the ground or turning too much. Ease off the stretch and repeat with less motion and you should feel a deep and relieving QL stretch. As with any stretching this can be repeated 3-4 times daily for 20-30 seconds until symptoms resolve. Once your symptoms resolve, this is a great stretch to perform daily after sitting, exercise or daily activities that may cause some back tightness.

Glute Stretches

The glutes are some of the most powerful muscles in the entire body so if they become tight and short they will restrict proper movement through the hip joints (remember these are the joints that should be creating movement, NOT the lumbar spine) and force the spine to move more which will in turn create lumbar strain, breakdown and pain. One of the easiest ways to stretch the glutes is simply sitting and doing the Figure 4 stretch. Sit in a comfortable chair (preferably not a soft chair), find a comfortable neutral position for your spine (pain free) and cross your right leg over your left knee. While keeping your lower back lordotic, bend forward through your hips NOT your back until you feel a nice deep glute stretch, now raise your left heel off of the ground. Hold this position for 20-30 seconds.

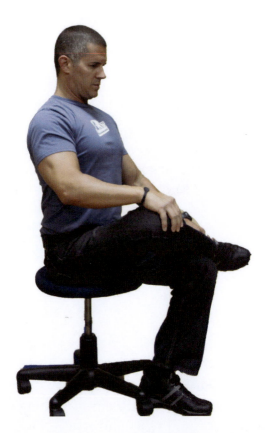

Seated Figure 4 Stretch. Note the neutral/lordotic lower back. NOT dropping the chest toward the knee (straining the lower back) or actively pressing the knee down (straining the front of the hip).

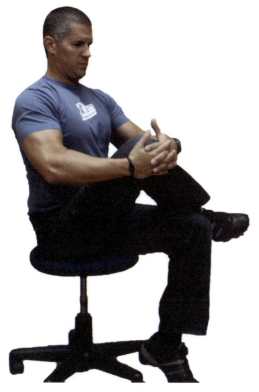

Seated Cross Glute Stretch. Note the neutral//lordotic lower back and no rotation/twisting of the lumbar spine. Simply raise the bottom leg heel off the ground and pull the knee to the opposite shoulder.

Now grab your right knee with your left hand and slowly pull it to your left shoulder. You should feel a different area of your right glute stretching. Hold this position for 20-30 seconds and repeat 2-3 times. If you feel any pain in the front of the hip or the knee, then simply adjust your position slightly (typically if you find a hybrid of the two stretches front hip or knee pain will resolve). Switch and do the left side 2-3 times and hold each stretch for 20-30 seconds. Remember to NEVER push down on your knee while doing the first Figure 4 stretch. This places the joint of the hip in a stressed position and can create irritation of the hip. Much like the Psoas and QL stretches, the glutes should be stretched after activity and should be used as a daily stretch to maintain healthy hips and healthy hip movement thus sparing the spine.

Cat/Camel Stretches

Now that we've unlocked those tight hypertonic muscles let's restore normal joint and nerve mobility to your spine with the Cat/Camel stretch. Assume a quadruped position with your hands under your shoulders and your knees under your hips.

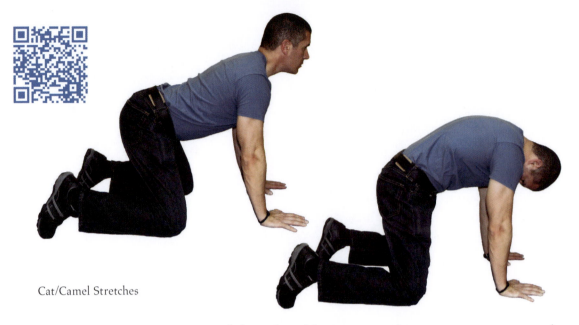

Cat/Camel Stretches

Now raise your spine up toward the ceiling like a cat stretching, as soon as you reach your greatest range of motion DON'T hold the position, immediately start to descend back to the bottom of the range like a camel back. Once at the bottom immediately return to the top and repeat 15-20 times until you feel nice and loose. Pain may be present at the top or bottom of this move, so you need to find a comfortable range of motion to follow. Go slowly and as you loosen up, gradually increase your range of motion. If discomfort or tightness completely abates after several repetitions (sometimes it will take 6-8 reps for this to happen) then continue with a full range of motion until you feel as though your spine is moving freely with no pain. It may take 15-20 repetitions for this pain free and stiffness free range of motion to occur. If the pain won't resolve at either the top or bottom of the range, then stop just short of the painful range and only perform the motion through that pain free range. Doing this move 3-4 times per day for 15-20 reps should start to free up those locked up joints and adhered nerves. Now you may be saying "But Dr. Rob you said never to flex the spine or you'll hurt your discs!!" Well you are correct! The one exception is the cat/camel. Because your spine has no load on it (the load of the upper body is on the hands) your discs are safe. Now, I would never recommend a Cat/Camel stretch for anyone with a flared up disc, that will just irritate it and potentially cause more of a bulge. But if the disc is no longer irritated or the pain is coming from a different area of the spine the cat/camel is a great move to regain spinal mobility as well as joint and nerve health. Once out of pain 2-3 sets of 10-20 reps of the Cat/Camel can be used daily as part of a healthy stretching routine to maintain good spinal mobility, nerve mobility and muscle flexibility.

**Quick Review: Proper Stretching for Extension Intolerant Lower Back Inuries**
**1. Psoas Stretches**
**2. Quadratus Lumborum (QL) Stretches**
**3. Glute Figure 4 Stretches**
**4. Cat/Camel Stretching**

Keep Your Spine in Mind

Once your pain has subsided significantly enough to resume normal activities of daily living make sure you continue to move throughout your day with your spine in mind. What I mean by that is protect your spine with neutral postures and hip hinging while bending forward and squeezing your glutes while reaching over-head.

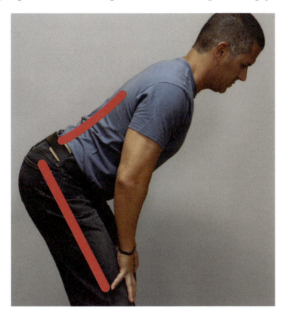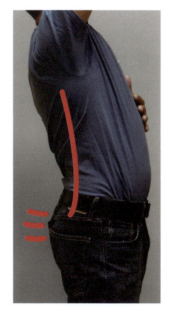

1. Leaning forward with a HIP HINGE (movement through the hips only) NOT the lower back. The lower back stays in a a neutral/lordotic position.
2. Leaning back with a GLUTE SQUEEZE and not hyper-extending the lower back.

By ensuring hip movement, not lumbar movement, the spine is spared and thus not aggravated. As general maintenance, I recommend doing the extension intolerance exercises 2-3 times per week to promote core strength and a healthy lower back. I also recommend performing the extension intolerance stretching daily, as a means to promote overall spinal and hip health. After a long day at work or after many hours of spring time yard work, a great time to stretch our hypertonic/short muscles is right before bed. A mere 2-3 minutes of stretching prior to bed is a great way to unwind tight muscles. As your body relaxes while sleeping, no strain is being placed on your musculoskeletal system so your bed time stretching routine will allow newly stretched muscles to stay relaxed so you can start your day with a more flexible and mobile muskuloskeletal system.

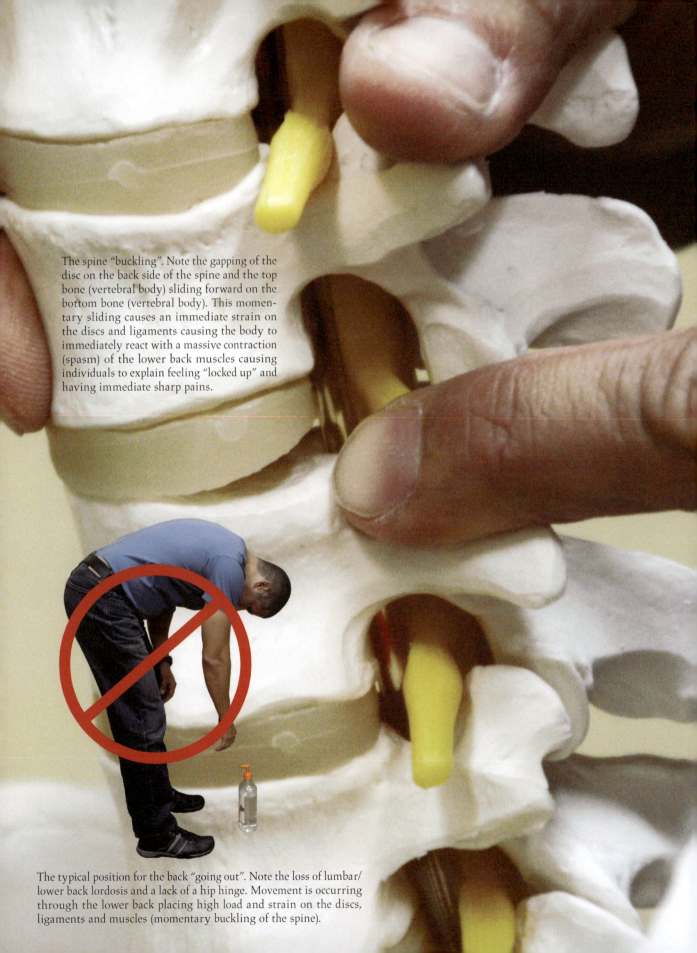

The spine "buckling". Note the gapping of the disc on the back side of the spine and the top bone (vertebral body) sliding forward on the bottom bone (vertebral body). This momentary sliding causes an immediate strain on the discs and ligaments causing the body to immediately react with a massive contraction (spasm) of the lower back muscles causing individuals to explain feeling "locked up" and having immediate sharp pains.

The typical position for the back "going out". Note the loss of lumbar/lower back lordosis and a lack of a hip hinge. Movement is occurring through the lower back placing high load and strain on the discs, ligaments and muscles (momentary buckling of the spine).

7

Easy Steps to Fix an Acute "MY BACK JUST WENT OUT" Episode of Back Pain

My Back Just Went Out! What Do I Do?

So here's the scenario, you're a chronic low back pain sufferer and have had a pretty good couple of months/weeks with your back not being irritated at all. Or, you've never had a back problem before. You're feeling good and don't think of your back at all as you bend forward without hip hinging and fully flex your low back to benignly pick up your sock off of the floor while you're getting ready for work. All of a sudden a sharp pain rips through your lower back! It's so sharp it takes your breath away as your muscles lock up in spasm! You're frozen and don't know what to do! You think "Oh No! I have to get the kids to school and then to work for that big meeting! What am I going to do? I can't move! I better start to stretch this spasm away!" STOP!!! The last thing you want to do is stretch a lumbar spine that has just spasmed. What happened was you placed your spine in a vulnerable position (forward bending/flexion) and it had no ability to stabilize itself. The muscles had no ability to hold the spine up in its lordosis (good curve) so the spine momentarily buckled. As a result the brain sent a massive contraction signal to the muscles in your spine to lock down the back muscles to prevent any more forward bending and thus buckling. This is purely a protective mechanism so you don't do catastrophic damage to your spine. Try bending forward while you're in an acute muscle spasm: you can't. Your brain won't allow it. It will create such intense pain and tightness you physically won't attempt to bend forward because it feels so terrible. Unfortunately, this exact measure of amelioration is what a lot of my patients do and are even taught to do by online "experts", fitness professionals and other health care providers. They are taught to lie on their backs and pull their knees to their chest and pull their knees across their body to stretch the pain away. I can't tell you how often I see this in clinical practice and I am here to tell you it is flat out *WRONG!!* When you are on your back and attempting to pull your knees to your chest you are creating lumbar flexion, the exact mechanism that caused the episode. So *STOP!* The first thing you are going to do is brace your core to keep your spine in a neutral position. Now gently get to the ground and lie on your stomach with your chin resting on your palms and let your entire body relax. After 1-2 minutes rise up so your chin is on your fists and completely relax. After another 1-2 minutes brace your core and raise up to a prone elbows position and hang out here for 2-3 minutes or longer and again, just relax (it may take 5 minutes or longer for the spasm to calm down).

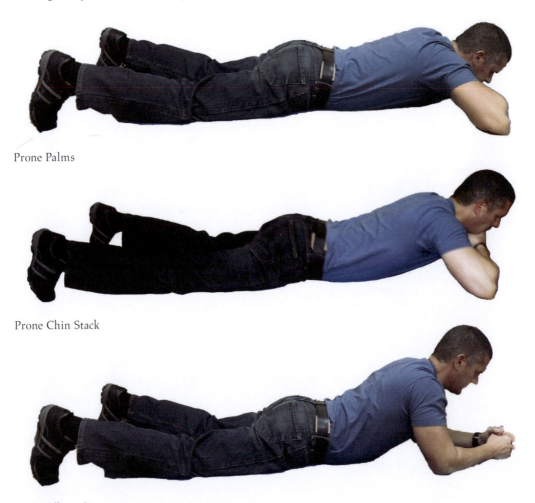

Prone Palms

Prone Chin Stack

Prone Elbows/Forearms

Now assume a push up position and do as many *Prone Lumbar Extension Presses* until you feel as though your back is relaxing, the spasms are diminishing and the pain is decreasing.

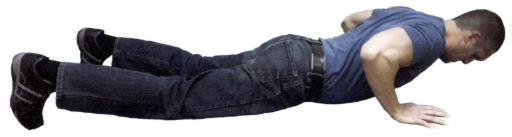

Start position of Prone Lumbar Extension Presses

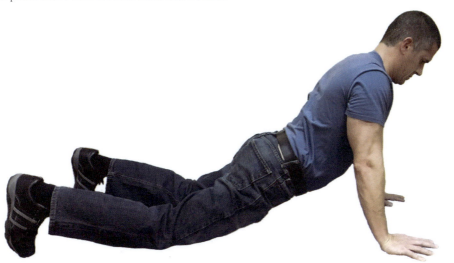

Finish position of Prone Lumbar Extension Presses

You may have to do 2-3 sets of 10-20 (or more) reps of *Prone Lumbar Extension Presses* with alternating resting periods on your elbows or in a chin fist stack before the acute spasms begin to relax. Once the spasms feel like they are starting to calm, brace your core, keep your spine in a neutral lordotic position and begin to rise from the ground. This should start with a quadruped position, then to kneeling, then to a lunge, then standing.

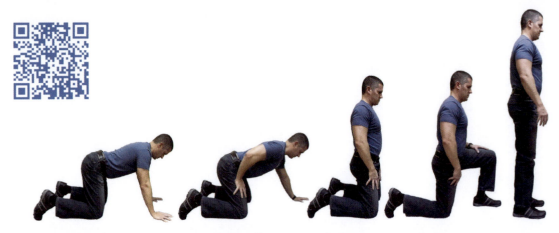
Getting up properly will ensure you don't restrain your back.

Move around and see how you feel. *DON'T BEND* to test your back, you'll just start a spasm cycle again! Moving very cautiously with spine sparing movement should also assist in calming the spasms in the lower back. Repeat the previous steps hourly (if needed) until the pain subsides. Once the pain is resolved (it may take several days) follow the protocols for lumbar flexion intolerance/disc based pain and you should recover quite quickly from this acute episode. Remember, the injury was caused by flexion of the spine, so take that move out of your repertoire of bending. Utilize the hip hinge to bend and your back won't go out!

> **Quick Review: If Your Back Just "Went Out" Do:**
> **1. Prone Lumbar Chin Stacks**
> **2. Prone Lumbar Elbows**
> **3. Prone Lumbar Extension Presses**

Proper Movement is the Key to a Pain Free Lower Back

If you take the previous several examples on what typically injuries the lower back, you'll find a consistent trend; improper movement and positioning is what typically causes injury. That's why I've been repeatedly teaching you to move through your hips while keeping your spine in a good lordotic neutral position. When analyzing power lifters, you can see they tend to be a great example of utilizing good stable

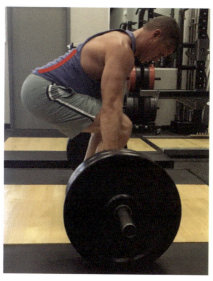

Note the good, safe neutral spine/lordosis that is kept during heavy lifting. Without this position the lifter could not achieve a powerful lift safely and can potentially cause serious lower back injury.

hip motion with a neutral lumbar spine. They use the techniques of lumbar neutral/lordosis and hip hinging to lift hundreds of pounds of weight (the world record in the squat lift is over 1000 pounds!!). If a power lifter flexed the spine with that much weight on his back, the results would be catastrophic injury. He'd end up in an ambulance on the way to the emergency room! So why aren't we doing this type of movement in everyday life? I'm not saying you need to become a power lifter and start lifting the back end of your car for fitness. I'm merely trying to change the paradigm of movement. We all become complacent over time and just dump our chest forward and round the lower back, in an unsafe position, dozens upon dozens of times throughout the day. If we would just take the time, learn these easy and safe movement patterns and simply apply them in everyday life, your back pain will start to diminish. If you keep your lordosis throughout activities of daily living your back will be protected, like a power-lifter's. As with individuals with flexion intolerance/disc pain, if moving through your hips with a neutral spine and utilizing the golfers pick up and the squat and lunge, your back will stay stable, it will heal and you can become an individual who doesn't have back pain. Yes, you read that correctly! If you make good sound movement choices the new normal and take out flexing the spine and twisting/rotation you can start to live a back pain free life! I see it every day in practice. Patients that have followed my protocols, and have learned to incorporate my movement techniques, actually become pain free and stay that way! You can too if you just commit to changing a few simple things.

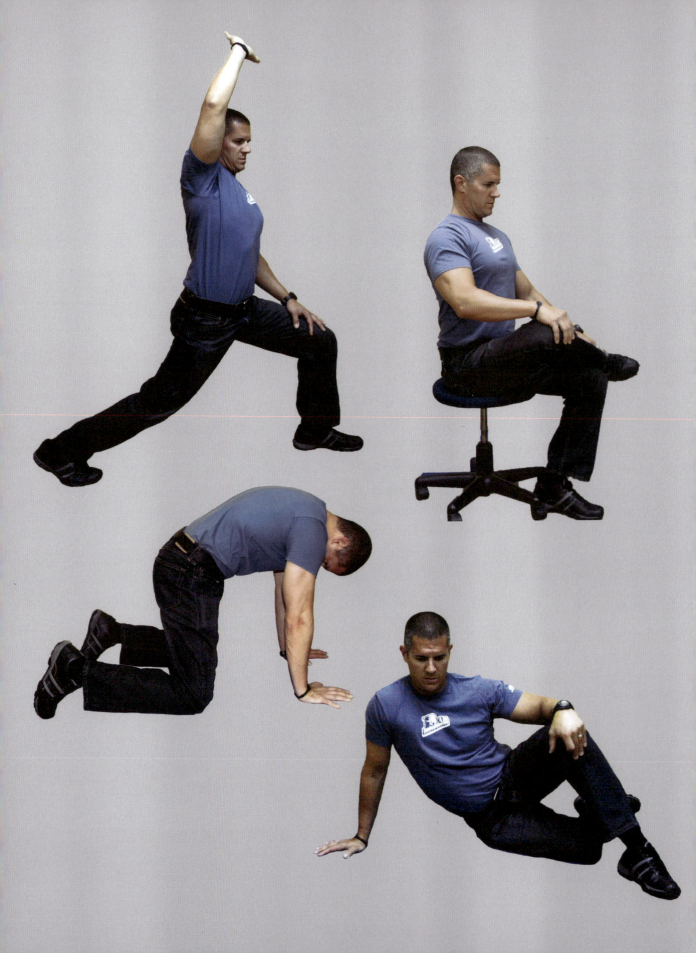

8

Easy Steps to Fix Back Stiffness

Simple Stretches for Back Stiffness

So here is a scenario that I see less often in my practice, but does exist. An individual has no discernable pain but has some back stiffness from chronically tight muscles, an old disc injury or maybe some mild arthritis. Again, the same rules apply, we don't place the spine under any risk by forward bending to stretch out the back. What I typically do for these patients is simply teach them how to move through their hips (hip hinging) while maintaining a neutral lumbar lordosis, so they don't cause any damage to their spines and become a pain sufferer. Next, a simple flexibility routine that includes Cat/Camel stretches, Side Lying QL stretches, Thoracic Rotations and Glute stretches and Psoas stretches to introduce mobility to joints that are immobile, safe stretching to muscles that are hypertonic (short and tight) and postural positions that are spine sparing. In fact, once an individual is out of either flexion intolerant/disc pain or extension intolerant pain these five stretches are a great way to cool down after a workout, loosen up the spine and hips after yard work or simply unwind before bed. I typically recommend stretching AFTER activity. Muscles will contract thousands of times during an exercise event, doing chores around the house or doing yard work. As a result, your muscles will tend to tighten up, so immediately after activity is a great time to perform these stretches. A daily routine of only 2-3 minutes will go a long way in keeping your spine in a good healthy state.

Quick Review: For Back Stiffness Do:
1. Psoas Stretches
2. Glute Stretches
3. QL Stretches
4. Cat/Camel Stretches
5. Thoracic Extensions/Rotation Stretches

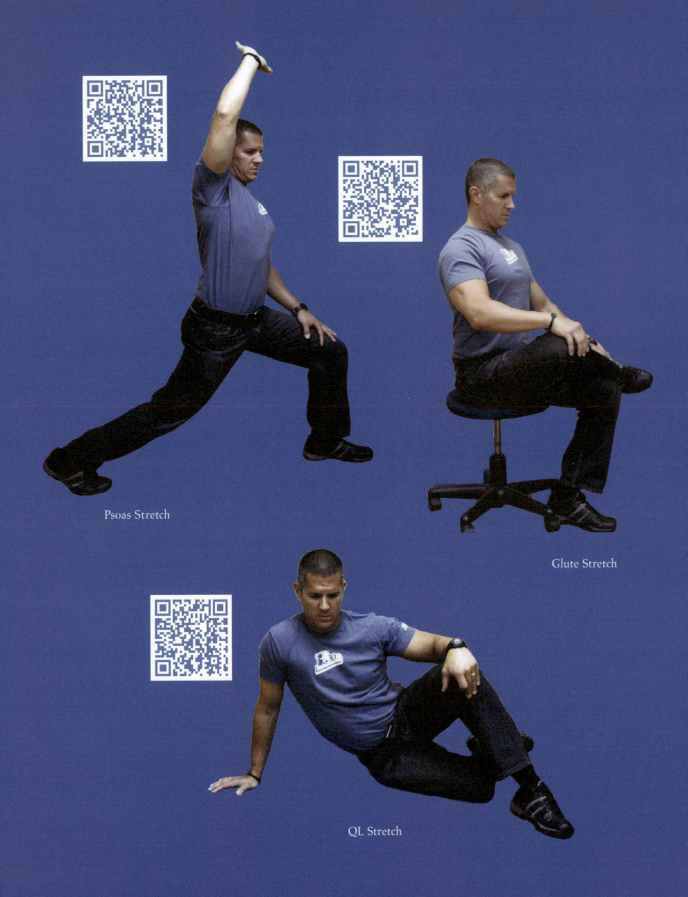

Psoas Stretch

Glute Stretch

QL Stretch

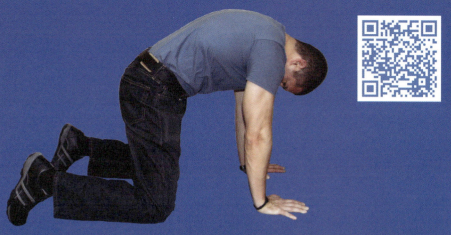

Cat/Camel Stretch

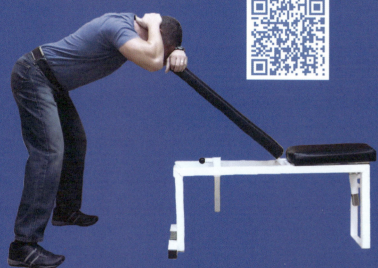

Thoracic Rotations

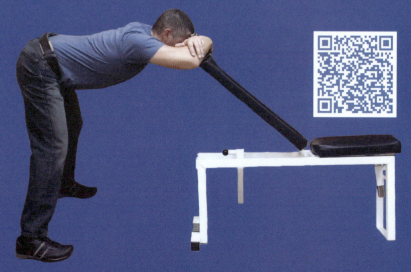

Thoracic Extensions

Back Breakers

Back Builders

9

Proper Core Work—Knowing How to Recognize Dr. Rob's "Back Breakers" and Dr. Rob's "Back/Core Builders"

SAFE Core Work Versus Injurious Core Work

So you've made it. You're out of back pain! Congratulations! Now it's time to build a strong core to protect your back. If you've taken the time to read the section on flexion intolerant/disc pain you should already know that if you *MOVE THE SPINE DURING EXERCISE YOU WILL BREAK IT DOWN.* But wait, "crunches, sit-ups, Russian twists, v-ups and hanging leg raises work my abs really hard. What am I supposed to do to build my core and abs?". I hear that question daily from patients that have been brain washed by the fitness industry to think that the only way to work the abs and build a strong core is to lie on your back or get into a pike position. I tell all my patients they may in fact work their abs by doing the "back breakers" but it's not a matter of *IF* they will hurt their backs but *WHEN!* So why even take the chance? The research is so clear on what actually injures the spine it infuriates me to know that so many fitness professionals and practitioners in the rehab and medical world are still being paid by unwitting individuals to end up injured! I've dealt with lower back pain myself for more than twenty years because nobody taught me how to move the proper way and exercise properly to spare my spine when I was young and impressionable. So let's stop the madness right here and right now and learn how to *PROPERLY* work the core and above all else *PROTECT YOUR BACK!*

How Back Breakers Injure the Spine

As I stated previously *if you are moving your spine to work the core you are breaking it down!* It's that simple! According to renowned physical therapist Grey Cook "The act of not moving during the presence of motion is true neuromuscular stabilization (true core training)". So right away, that takes the vast majority of "ab" exercises off the "Back/Core Builders" list and places them on the "Back Breakers" list.

Dr. Rob's Back Breakers—Warning: Don't Do These!

Sit-ups	Supermans/extensions
Russian twists	Hyper extensions from a bench
Crunches	Knee raises from hanging
Bicycle crunches	abdominal board
Oblique crunches	Lying knees to chest
V sits	Crunches on a ball
V ups	Side lying crunches
Deep Squats	Side lying sit ups
Toe touches	Not maintaining Lordosis
Burpees	during a dead lift or squat

Traditional moves that I believe are being epidemically taught in fitness clubs, aerobic classes, body "blasting" classes and in some Pilates studios are breaking many of the rules with regard to how the core works. The ultimate job of the core is to *STOP MOTION OF THE SPINE IN THE PRESENCE OF MOTION.* So what does this mean? In the simplest of terms, it means the muscles of the core stabilize the spine from moving (keeping it stable and rigid) while motion is being created by the ball and socket joints of the hips and shoulders. So if you take Dr. Rob's number one "back breaker" the Sit-Up and analyze its motion, it's breaking the cardinal rules of the core. The Sit-Up creates flexion motion in the spine with the abs and the hip flexors. Dr. Rob's number two "back breaker" the Russian Twist is breaking the same basic rule, its creating spinal motion around the lumbar spine in the form of rotation (a movement that is great at creating disc issues in the low back!). Again, the hips are supposed to be creating motion and the core is supposed to be stopping the spine from moving. Both the sit-up and the Russian Twist create motion through the spine with core muscles. If you want to create a nice big disc herniation I recommend doing lots of sit-ups and Russian twists! If you want to protect your back, I recommend *NEVER DOING THEM!!*

I could go on and on about all of the "back breaker" exercises but in the interest of boring you to death with the details of why they are bad just remember the simple fact that *they move the spine during exercise and as a result break it down.*

Back Breaker Exercises do the following:

1. <u>Flex the Spine</u>—for example: touching your toes, doing a sit up/crunch, deep squatting or deadlifting while not maintaining lumbar lordosis throughout the entirety of the movement.
2. <u>Rotate the Spine</u>—for example: Russian twists, "oblique" crunches, rotational stretching
3. <u>Put the Spine Under Load</u>—for example: seated crunches, weighted crunches or sit-ups and weighted Russian twists.
4. <u>Any Combination of the above</u>—for example: burpees, Russian twists, Sit ups with twists

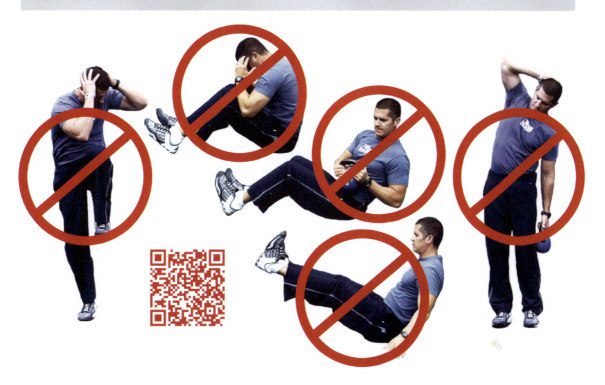

Dr. Rob's Back Breakers for Core Exercise

Please remember that the "back breakers" will almost always: flex the spine, twist/rotate the spine, place the spine under load and move the spine through a range of motion. All of these activities have potential to cause damage to the joints, discs, ligaments and nerves of your lower back. Please avoid ALL of these moves at all cost. Unfortunately the world of exercise and fitness are constantly trying to come up with the latest and greatest moves for a strong core and an overall stronger body often to the detriment of the spine. Because there are so many bad moves I can't list them herein but what I can tell you is scrutinize an exercise that you are suspicious about; does it flex the spine? Does it rotate the spine? Does it take the spine through a range of motion? If it does any of these then you know it has potential to hurt your back and cause you pain. So STOP DON'T DO IT! If you are in a group fitness class, watching an exercise DVD or simply using the exercises a magazine is recommending for "chiseled abs by next summer" and you think one or many of the exercises are potentially detrimental to your lower back simply substitute a "back breaker" with one of Dr. Rob's "core/back builders".

Proper Core Training—The Basics

So, now that I've hopefully convinced you to NOT do the "back breakers" which exercises remain to build a good strong core? Well, the answer is a lot! Remember the core's job is to stabilize the spine while the hips and shoulders are moving through a range of motion. So the "back/core builders" I recommend to my back pain patients and to the athletes I train will encompass varying levels of difficulty while always being mindful of prioritizing the spine. Some are performed on the ground and some are performed while standing so patients can learn to stabilize their spines while they are performing activities of daily living. We don't spend our days lying on our backs so why would we just do our core work lying down?

STOP Pulling Your Belly Button Back to Your Spine to Contract Your Core!

Before we get into the safe ways to create a strong core and a healthy spine I would like to quickly address two issues that continue to plague my patients and potentially, you as well. When a true core "brace" or core contraction is applied by an individual (I will fully explain how to do this shortly) the muscles of the core stiffen to create a muscular corset around the spine. This can only be accomplished by bracing as if you are going to be punched in the belly and *ALL* the muscles of your mid-section contract as one unit. I have to retrain many of my back pain patients out of the habit of belly button sucking/vacuuming as a core brace technique. Many fitness instructors, physical therapists and Pilates instructors will teach individuals to suck the belly button in while attempting to core brace for exercise. This is not only flat out wrong it's dangerous to the health of your spine! As renowned researcher Stuart McGill states "the act of pulling the belly button back toward the spine to stabilize the core is a "myth". When this move is attempted by individuals to brace their cores, they are actually *destabilizing* the spine by only contracting a small amount of musculature namely the transverse abdominus. Please remember, while doing ANY core work or any movement that requires abdominal bracing *DON'T PULL YOUR BELLY BUTTON BACK TO YOUR SPINE!*

NEVER Press Your Lower Back to the Floor for "Support"

Similar to the misinformation about belly button sucking in to brace the core, is the act of pressing your low back into the floor while doing core work. The act of keeping the lumbar spine in a neutral position, usually with a degree of lordosis has been a consistent theme through the entirety of this book. Lumbar lordosis is the most stable, and safe position for the lower back, as it is designed to handle the greatest amount of load from this position. Remember, if the lumbar spine is in flexion it can't handle load and will break the discs down. Well, guess what happens when you are lying on your back and you press your low back into the floor to "stabilize it"? You place it into flexion! A position that can't carry load! Picture this, your fitness trainer or exercise DVD has instructed you to get on your back. While in this position, you've pressed your lower back into the ground to "stabilize" it. Now, you repeatedly flex it over and over and over again while you perform crunches, sit ups, v-ups and other "back breakers". Yes, you've worked your abs slightly, but guess what? You've basically been pumping your discs out from their normal position and progressed yourself towards a nice big painful disc bulge! You should now understand the potential for disc injury as the spine is flexed while performing exercise. So please, if you want to have a healthy lower back, *DON'T PRESS YOUR LOWER BACK TO THE FLOOR!*

How to Perform a PROPER Core/Abdominal Brace

Alright, now that we know the perils of belly button vacuuming and pressing the low back to the floor, let's learn how to do a proper core set/abdominal brace. Believe it or not, a true core set comes from the neck and works its way all the way down to the abdominals, and if standing, the glutes are also involved. Let's start on our backs for the *Dying Bug*. 1. Pack your neck as if you are giving yourself a double chin. 2. Raise your chest up by pulling your shoulder blades back and down like they are being placed into your back pockets. 3. Most importantly, brace your abdominals like someone is going to punch or kick you in the side or stomach and you have to protect your organs (you should feel as though your entire mid-section pushed outwards, as if you were trying to fill the empty space between your midsection and an imaginary belt that was wrapped around you).

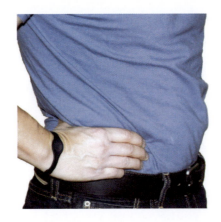

Again, don't suck your belly button back to your spine! If you are having trouble feeling this stand up and place your fingers into your stomach and your thumbs into your lower back, now cough vigorously. You should feel your core muscles push out against your fingers and thumbs. Now do this again, but this time hold the muscle contraction after the cough and you will feel what it's like to have a true core set/abdominal brace.

So now that you know how to truly brace your core and place your spine in a good safe position let's start with core work on the floor:

The following exercises are safe and healthy for your back IF DONE PROPERLY. They are labelled for progression as (B) BASIC, (I) INTERMEDIATE and (A) ADVANCED. If you feel any strain or pain DO NOT ADVANCE. Stay with and master the Basic (B) exercises before moving on to the Intermediate (I) and Advanced (A) exercises. Each grouping of exercises are labelled with (B), (I) and (A) so PROPER PROGRESSION can be made. This is very important simply because core bracing and form are paramount to doing perfect core exercise. Remember pain should ALWAYS be your guideline. Don't rush these exercises. Master each level before advancing for a strong and stable core and a healthy back. And always remember, DON'T LET GO OF YOUR CORE BRACE THROUGHOUT THE ENTIRETY OF EACH AND EVERY REP OF EACH EXERCISE!! True core stability is attained by not just having a strong core but a core that has good endurance. That means the ability to maintain a core brace while breathing (this is more challenging than one would think!) during exercise and while performing activities of daily living.

Dr. Rob's Core/Back Builders:

Unlike the "back breakers" Dr. Rob's "core/back builders" follow a couple of very simple rules that I've talked about consistently throughout this entire book. 1. They NEVER flex the spine. 2. They NEVER rotate the spine. 3. They NEVER move the spine through a range of motion. What my "core/back builders" do is create core stability and strength by bracing the core musculature, locking the spine into a safe position and only moving the ball and socket joints. Research shows that the endurance of the core musculature (how long the muscles can perform before fatiguing) is the most important component for full back protection. As such hold times and increases of repetitions are how my "core/back builders" will progress. Building a strong core to protect your back is not about how strong your core is so you can lift a heavy object once; it's about the continued contraction of the core muscles to ensure a stabilized and protected spine during activities that are prolonged. As you fatigue the core musculature must have good endurance capacity or risk of injury is greatly increased.

The following list may seem extensive but there are actually many more safe moves that I do myself and recommend to my patients. For a complete list with many options for all levels of strength and fitness please check out my website protectyourback101.com. Due to the varying degrees of difficulty of these exercises and the different levels of fitness that we all have I will list beginner (B), intermediate (I) and advanced (A) with each exercise. As part of a sound core building program these exercises can be performed 5-6 times per week to build a strong core or 2-3 times per week to maintain core endurance, strength and stability. Each exercise should be performed for 2-3 sets. Remember, all exercises are not for all people. If an exercise doesn't feel right or it hurts a knee, wrist or shoulder simply move on to the next progression. Because there are so many exercises listed and in attempt to not confuse or overwhelm you a good rule of thumb to follow is choose 1-2 exercises from 3 or 4 sections and do 2-3 sets of each. The next workout session you have the next day or later in the week choose another 1-2 exercises per section and do 2-3 sets of each. Please progress smartly and conservatively. If you follow my recommendations you can and will achieve a good strong core and a pain free back. Enjoy your workout and most important of all Protect Your Back!

1. Bird Dog Progressions

(B) Basic Bird Dog

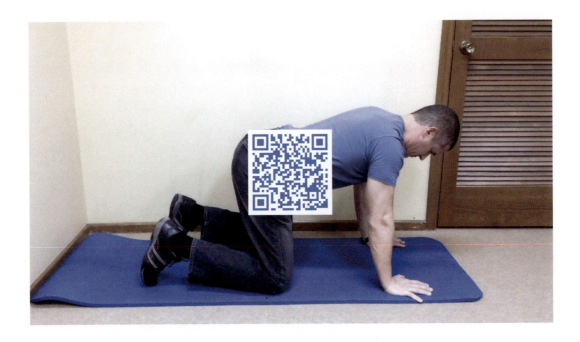

As with all core work ensure a neutral/lordotic low back position. This should be a position that is pain free and for the bird dog you should be able to balance a tennis ball on the small of your back without it rolling off through the entire movement. If you can do this you'll know your spine hasn't moved and only the ball and socket joints of the shoulder and hips have. Brace your core, slowly elevate your right arm and left leg back until they are parallel to the ground. Hold it for 5 seconds. Return it slowly and controlled to the start position and repeat with your opposite arm and leg. Aim for 10 repetitions on each side with a 5 second hold each. If you are too fatigued and you cannot hold form then simply hold the position for less time. Once you can do 10 repetitions per side for a 10 second hold each you are ready to advance to the next move.

(B) <u>Bird Dog with Sweeps</u>

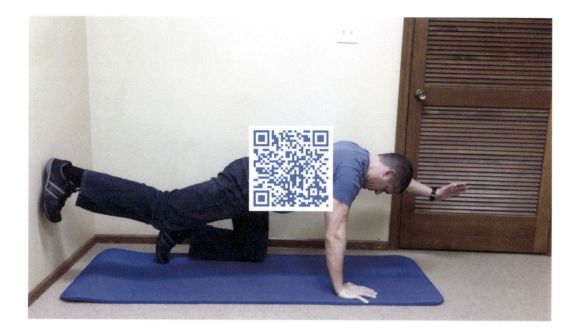

Start as per the basic bird dog but instead of lowering the arm and leg to the ground and switching to the opposite side after raising use the same arm and leg to sweep the ground and return the arm and leg to a parallel to the floor position. Hold for 5 seconds again and do 5 total sweeps on that same side. Now repeat on the opposite side. Once you can perform 10 sweeps with 10 seconds hold each rep per side you are ready to advance to the next exercise.

(I) Bird Dog with Circles or Squares

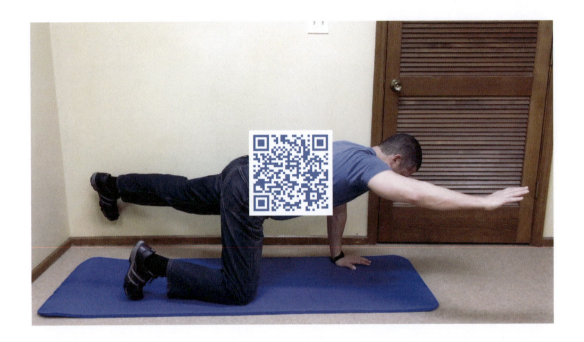

Start as per the basic bird dog but at the fully extended position hold the arm and leg out and perform 5 air circles or squares, switch to the opposite side and repeat 5 circles or squares. Once you can perform 5 reps per side of 10 air squares or circles you are ready to advance to the Bear.

2. Bear Progressions

(B) Basic Bear

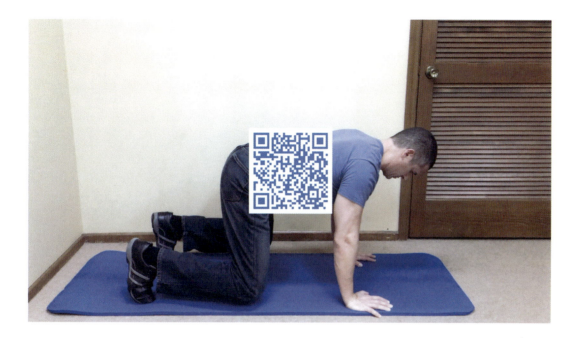

From a quadruped position with hands under shoulders and knees under hips ensure your spine is in a good pain free lordosis. Retract (pull your shoulder blades together and down—into your back pockets), pack your neck and brace your core. Now raise your knees off the ground only 3-5 inches. Ensure your lumbar spine did not move. Now hold this position for 5 seconds. Repeat 5 repetitions. Once you can perform 10 repetitions with 10 second holds each you are ready to progress to the Bear March.

(I) Bear March

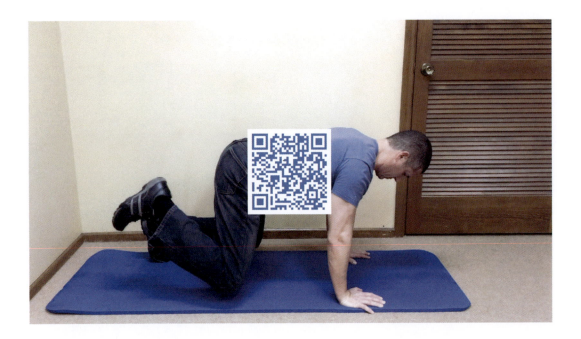

Start exactly as the basic bear and raise your knees 3-5 inches off of the ground. Now hold this position for 5 seconds as with the basic bear. After 5 seconds don't lower to the ground, raise your right foot so you are only balancing on the left and hold for 5 seconds, set your right foot down now immediately raise your left foot and hold for 5 seconds. Repeat 5 total reps. Once you can progress to and perform 10 reps of each for 10 seconds you are ready to progress to the Bear Arm Raise.

(I) Bear Arm Raise

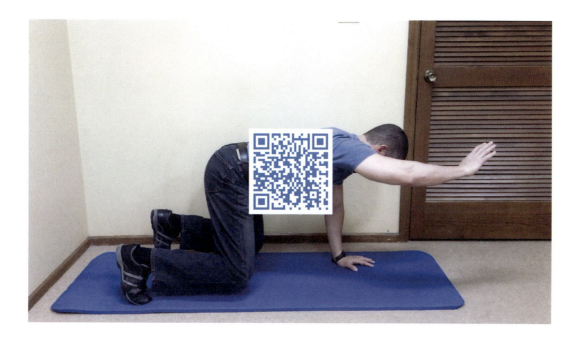

Start exactly as the basic bear and raise your knees 3-5 inches off of the ground. Now Brace your core hard and squeeze your shoulder blades together to brace your upper body. Lean slightly to your left without moving your spine and raise your right arm up like you're flying like Superman. Hold for 5 seconds then repeat on left side. That's one rep. Do 5 total per side and see how you feel. If it was quite hard then 5 reps of 5 seconds should be your starting point. Your goal should be 10 reps per side with a 10 second hold each. Once you can master this move you're ready for the Bear Donkey Kick.

(A) Bear Donkey Kick

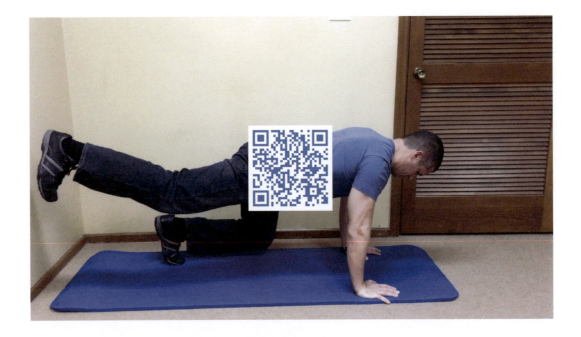

Start exactly as the basic bear and raise your knees 3-5 inches off the ground. Now brace your core hard and squeeze your shoulder blades together as you kick your right leg straight back until your leg is parallel to the ground. Hold this for 5 seconds and repeat on the left side. Once you can do 10 reps per side with 10 seconds holds you are ready to advance to the Bear Around the World.

(A) Bear Around the World

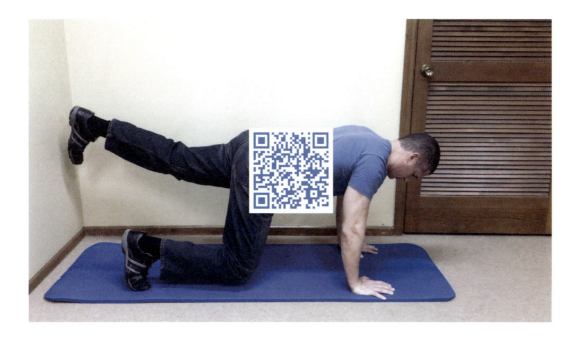

Start exactly as the basic bear and raise your knees 3-5 inches off the ground. Now brace your core and squeeze your shoulder blades together. Raise your left leg and hold for 5 seconds, now raise your right leg and hold for 5 seconds, now slightly lean to your left and raise your right arm up and hold for 5 seconds then lower your arm and slightly lean to your right and raise your left arm for 5 seconds; all without lowering your knees to the ground. That is 1 rep. When you can perform 10 reps each for 10 seconds holds you are ready to progress to the Bear Bird Dog.

(A) Bear Bird Dog

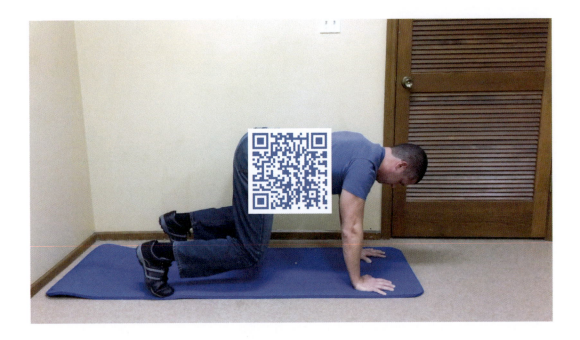

Start exactly as the basic bear and raise your knees 3-5 inches off the ground. Now brace your core hard and squeeze your shoulder blades together as you kick your right leg straight back and your left arm straight forward until they are parallel to the ground. Hold for 5 seconds and repeat with the left leg and right arm. If you can perform 10 reps per side of 10 seconds each you have a very strong, stable core and great balance!

3. Plank Progressions

(B) Basic Elbow Plank

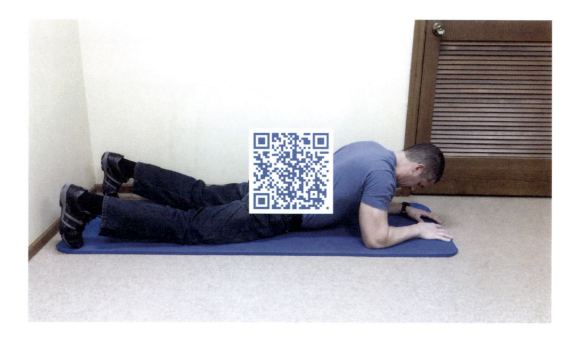

Start by lying on your stomach with your elbows propped under your shoulders. Brace your core and raise your body up until only your toes and elbows are on the ground. Don't look up; pick a spot on the ground so your neck stays packed. Now hold this position until you start to shake and feel like you can't keep your core braced and spine supported. Holding a plank for excessive time while your shaking like crazy won't do you any good; you'll be letting go of your core brace and not properly stabilizing the spine. DON'T HOLD YOUR BREATH! Breathe normally. Once you feel like you can't sustain a braced core lower yourself to the ground and check your time. If it was less than 20 seconds you should perform 4-5 reps of 20 second planks for 2-3 sets. Once you can hold your plank for 30 seconds perform 3-4 reps of 30 second planks for 2-3 sets. Once you can hold your plank for 1 minute or more do 2-3 sets of 1 minute planks. Once you can achieve a 1 minute plank for 2-3 sets you are ready to advance to Planks with Pulses.

(I) Plank with Pulses

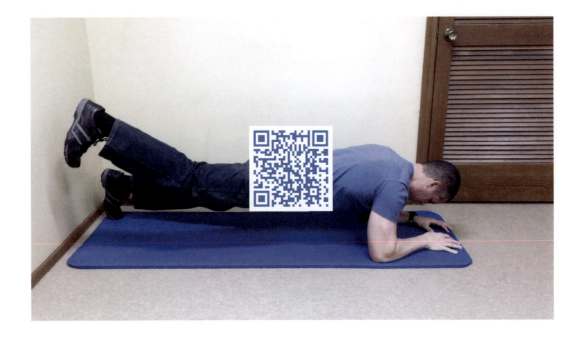

Start as per the basic plank. Brace your core and raise your body up until only your toes and elbows are on the ground. Now raise your right leg up until you feel your right glute contract (not too high, we don't want the spine to move) then lower it back to the ground and tap your toe. Immediately raise your right leg back up and repeat 5 times. Switch to the left side without lowering your body to the ground and do 5 pulses. Do a total of 5 reps per side with 5 pulses each. Once you can perform 10 reps per side with 10 pulses each you are ready to progress to the Plank Donkey Kick.

(I) Plank Donkey Kicks

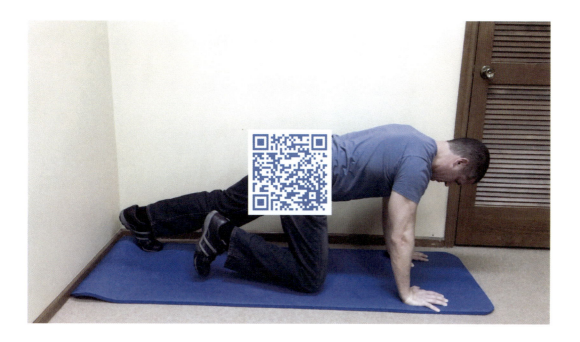

Start as per the basic plank but from a pushup position. Brace your core and raise your body up until only your toes and hands are on the ground. Now bring your right leg toward your chest until your hip is bent 90 degrees. DON'T take it higher than 90 degrees; if you do you will flex your spine and place pressure on the discs. Now kick your right leg back until it is parallel to the ground and you feel your glute contract. Do 5 Donkey Kicks then repeat on the left side. Do 5 donkey kicks per side for 5 reps each. Once you can perform 10 reps per side of 10 donkey kicks each leg you are ready to progress to Plank Shoulder Touches.

(I) Plank Shoulder Touches

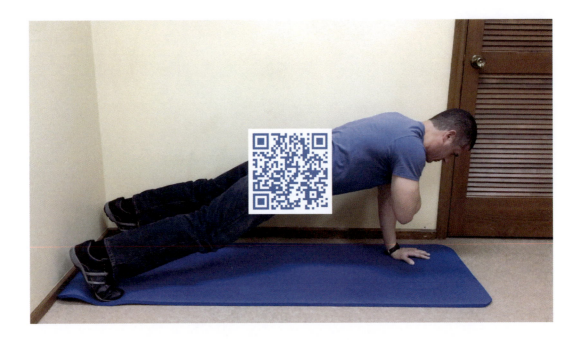

    Start as per the basic plank but from a pushup position. Brace your core and raise your body up until only your toes and hands are on the ground. Now squeeze your shoulder blades together and lean slightly to your left side. Touch your left shoulder with your right hand 5 times then repeat on your left side. That's 1 rep. Do 5 reps total per side with 5 shoulder touches. Once you can perform 3-4 reps per side of 10 shoulder touches you are ready to progress to the Plank Around the World.

(A) Plank Around the World

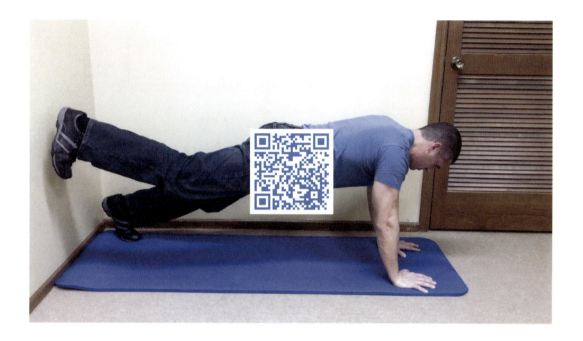

Start as per the basic plank but from a pushup position. Brace your core and raise your body up until only your toes and hands are on the ground. Now raise your right leg off the ground until it is parallel to the ground and hold it there for 5 seconds, lower it to the start position and raise your left leg off the ground and hold for 5 seconds. Lower it and raise your left arm off the ground and hold for 5 seconds, lower it and now raise your right arm off the ground for 5 seconds. Lower your body to the ground and rest for 2 seconds. That's 1 rep. Do 5 reps in total for 5 seconds each. Once you can perform 10 reps around the world with 10 seconds hold each limb you are ready to advance to the Elbow Plank Lat Row and the Push-Up Planks Lat Row.

(A) Elbow Plank Lat Rows

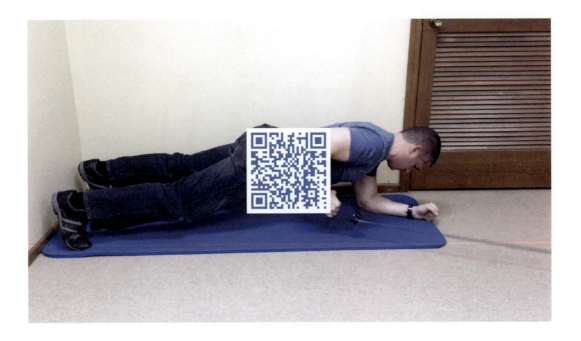

Start as per the basic plank. Brace your core and raise your body up until only your toes and elbows are on the ground. Firmly grab the handle of a connected band or pully with your right hand and simply pull until your hand is at the bottom of your rib cage. There should be no spinal motion or torso twisting. Make sure you set your shoulder blades and look at the ground NOT up (to ensure you are not straining your neck). Do 5 reps then switch to your left side. Your goal should be 10-15 reps of lat rows per side for 3 total sets per side. Once you can perform 10-15 reps per side for 3 sets you are ready to progress to the Push Up Plank Lat Row.

(A) Pushup Plank Lat Row

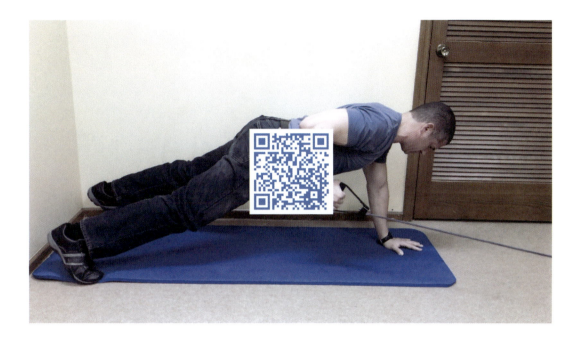

Start as per the basic plank but from a pushup position. Brace your core and firmly grab the handle of a connected band or pully with your right hand and simply pull until your hand is at the bottom of your rib cage. There should be no spinal motion or torso twisting. Make sure you set your shoulder blades and look at the ground NOT up (to ensure you are not straining your neck). Do 5 reps then switch to your left side. Your goal should be 10-15 reps of lat rows per side for 3 total sets per side. Once you can achieve 10-15 reps of lat rows per side for 3 sets you are ready to progress to the most advanced planks; Ball Roll Outs, Ball Shoulder Circles and the Ab Wheel.

(A) Ball Shoulder Circles

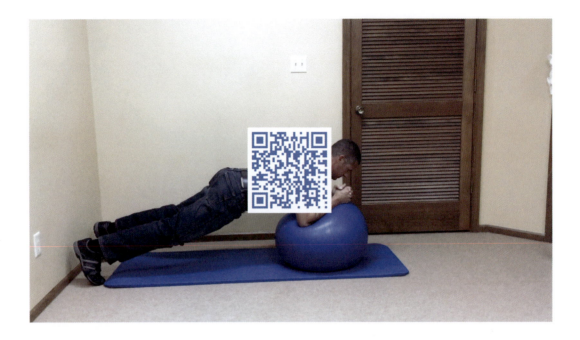

From a full plank position brace your core, pack your neck and squeeze your shoulder blades together while your elbows are on a fit ball under your shoulders. While maintaining this set position slowly roll your SHOULDERS ONLY in a circular position. The key to this move as with all planks is to KEEP YOUR SPINE STILL, there should be no movement anywhere except the shoulders. Remember to NEVER LET GO OF YOUR CORE throughout the ENTIRETY OF THIS MOVEMENT. Do 5 circles in a clockwise direction, then 5 circles in the counter-clockwise direction. Rest and repeat for 3 sets. Your goal should be 10 circles in each direction for 3 sets. To make this move more difficult you can extend your elbows further out and perform the circles.*

*Please note the last three moves are quite challenging and with all of our exercises if performed properly there is no risk of injury (unlike Dr. Rob's Back Breakers that WILL injure you if you do them enough!). However if you are too fatigued and cannot brace your core properly you are risking possible back strain. Please listen to your body and if you are fatigued and cannot maintain a core brace throughout the ENTIRETY of the exercise please take a short rest then continue.

(A) Ball Rollouts

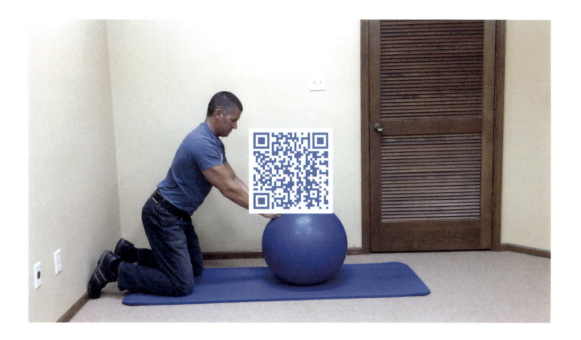

From a knee plank position on a ball brace your core, pack your neck and set your shoulder blades. Your elbows should be directly below your shoulders. With your core braced firmly slowly roll your elbows forward away from your body. Now with your core still braced, roll back to the starting position. Remember to NEVER LET GO OF YOUR CORE throughout the ENTIRETY OF THIS MOVEMENT. If you feel strain on your lower back STOP and don't go any further! Only work in a pain free range of motion. If there is some strain or pain you may not be ready for this move. If you feel weak don't extend your elbows out as far. If there is no pain/strain then do 5 reps of 5 seconds rolling out and 5 seconds rolling in for 3 sets. Your goal should be 10 reps of 5 seconds rolling out and back in for 3 sets.

(A) Ab Wheel

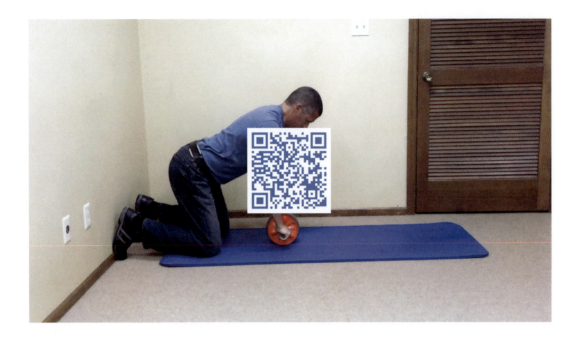

From a quadruped position, holding on to an ab wheel brace your core, pack your neck and set your shoulder blades. Firmly grasp the wheel handles. With your core braced slowly roll the wheel away from your body for a 5 second count then roll it back to the starting position for a 5 count. Remember to NEVER LET GO OF YOUR CORE throughout the ENTIRETY OF THIS MOVEMENT. If you feel strain on your lower back STOP and don't go any further! Only work in a pain free range of motion. If there is some strain or pain you may not be ready for this move. If you feel weak don't extend the wheel out as far. If there is no pain/strain then do 5 reps of 5 seconds rolling out and 5 seconds rolling back in for 3 sets. Your goal should be 10 reps of 5 seconds rolling out and back in for 3 sets.

(A) Plank Tricep Extension

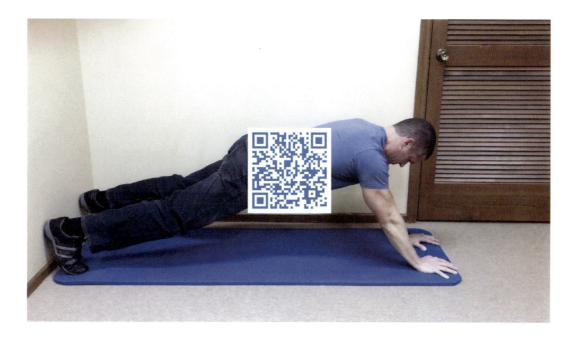

Start from an elbow plank position. Brace your core hard and drive your hands into the ground until you are up on your hands in a push up position. With a continued core brace lower yourself down back to your elbows. That's 1 rep. Now repeat until your arms and core are fatigued. Remember, this is an advanced move so be sure you can maintain a good strong core brace through the entirety of the movement.

(A) Plank Up Down

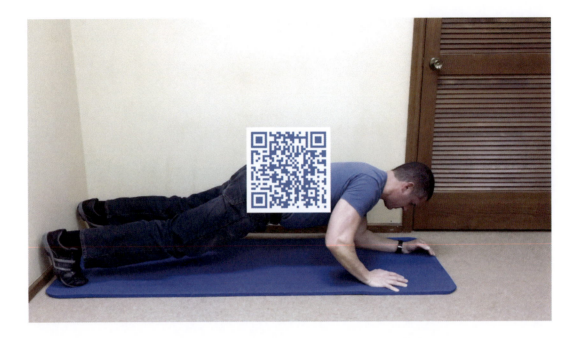

Start from an elbow plank position. Brace your core hard and place your right palm on the ground as if you are about to do a pushup, now place your left palm on the ground as if you are going to do a push up. Push your body up until you are in push-up plank position. Continue your strong core brace and lower yourself back to the starting position. That is 1 rep. Repeat until you are fatigued. Remember, this is an advanced move so be sure you can maintain a good strong core brace through the entirety of the movement.

4. Side Plank Progressions

(B) Side Lying Double Leg Raise

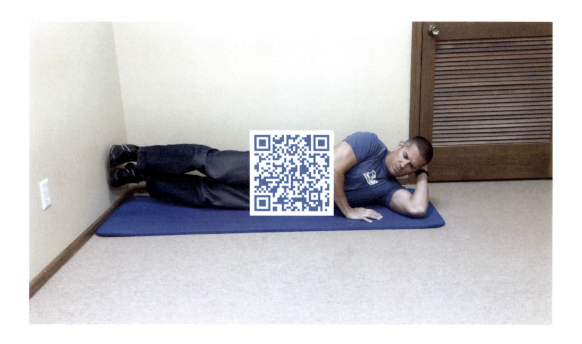

While lying on your left side, support your head with your down side arm. Be sure to keep your body perpendicular to the ground. Brace your core hard and raise both your top and bottom legs off of the ground. Now hold for 5-10 seconds. While maintaining your core brace lower your legs back to the ground. That's 1 rep. Do 5-6 reps with a goal of 10 reps per side with 10 seconds hold each. Remember, keep your core braced through the entirety of the movement. Once you can perform 10 reps per side with 10 seconds holds you are ready to progress to the ½ Side Bridge.

(B) Half Side Bridge

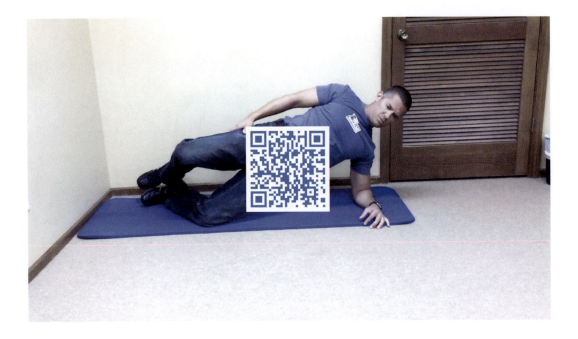

From a side lying position place your left elbow under your shoulder and your knees stacked in a position that is ahead of your hips by about 12 inches. Brace your core, raise your spine slightly so it is straight (you don't want to start this position with a sagging spine), squeeze your shoulder blades together and pack your neck. Now raise your hips off the ground by driving your down sided (left) knee into the ground while simultaneously raising or "clamming" your top leg, now push your hips forward until your abs and quads are lined up. Hold this position for 5 seconds. You should feel your down side glute and down side obliques and QL working really hard. Maintain this exact position until your left side is back to the ground, now you can relax for a second. Get set the EXACT same way for every rep until you do 5 reps per side with a 5 second hold. Your goal should be to do 10 reps per side with a 10 second hold each rep for 3 sets. If you have pain in your shoulder, back or neck STOP and reset your position. Even my patients with back and/or shoulder pain typically can find a pain free position if they stop and reset. Once you can do this you are ready to progress to the Half Side Bridge with Leg Raise.

(I) Half Side Bridge with Leg Raise

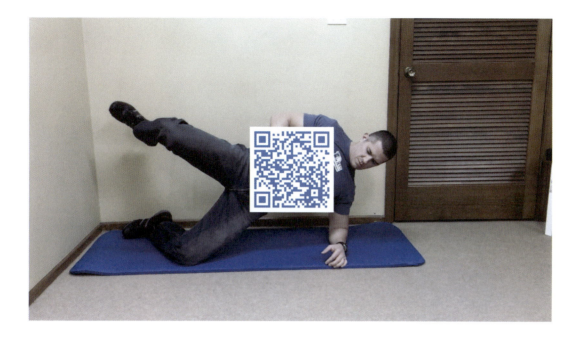

From a side lying position place your left elbow under your shoulder and your knees stacked in a position that is ahead of your hips by about 12 inches. Brace your core, raise your spine slightly so it is straight (you don't want to start this position with a sagging spine), squeeze your shoulder blades together and pack your neck. Now raise your hips off the ground while simultaneously raising your top leg while it is straight and push your hips forward until your abs and quads are lined up. While maintaining your core brace raise your top leg in a clamming fashion for 5 reps. Lower your body to the ground and repeat 3 more ½ Side Bridges up with 5 leg raises each. Once you've completed 4 reps of ½ Side Bridges with 5 clams each turn over to the other side and repeat. You should perform 2-3 sets each side. Your goal should be 6 reps of 6 leg raises each per side for 2-3 sets. Once you can do this you are ready to progress to the Full Side Plank.

(I) Full Side Bridge/Plank

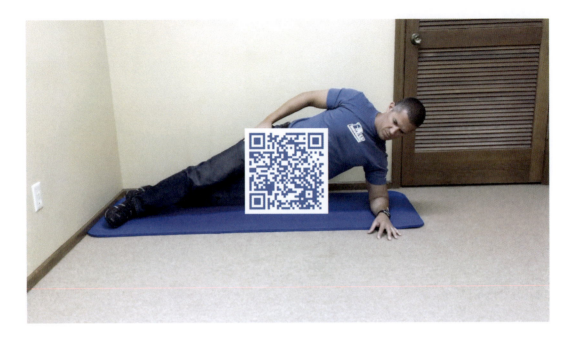

From a side lying position place your left elbow under your shoulder and your top foot (right) about 6 inches in front of your bottom (left) foot. By splitting your stance like this you will have better stability to hold the side plank. Brace your core, raise your spine slightly so it is straight (you don't want to start this position with a sagging spine), squeeze your shoulder blades together and pack your neck. Now raise your hips off the ground while pushing them forward. You should feel your down side glute and down side obliques and QL working really hard. Now hold this position until you start to shake and feel like you can't keep your core braced and spine supported. Holding a plank for excessive time while your shaking like crazy won't do you any good; you'll be letting go of your core brace and not properly stabilizing the spine. DON'T HOLD YOUR BREATH! Breathe normally. Once you feel like you can't sustain a braced core lower yourself to the ground (don't let go of your core brace until you are on the ground!) and check your time. If it was less than 20 seconds you should perform 4-5 reps of 20 second planks for 2-3 sets per side. Once you can hold your plank for 30 seconds perform 3-4 reps of 30 second planks for 2-3 sets. Once you can hold your plank for 1 minute or more on both sides do 2-3 sets of 1 minute planks. Once you can achieve a 1 minute plank for 2-3 sets you are ready to advance to the Full Side Plank with Leg Raise.

(A) Full Side Bridge/Plank with Leg Raise

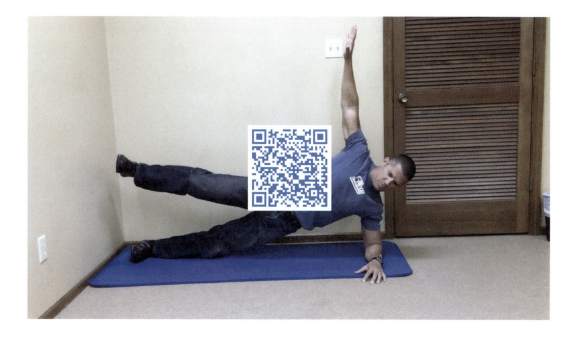

From a side lying position place your left elbow under your shoulder and your top foot (right) about 6 inches in front of your bottom (left) foot. By splitting your stance like this you will have better stability to hold the side plank. Brace your core, raise your spine slightly so it is straight (you don't want to start this position with a sagging spine), squeeze your shoulder blades together and pack your neck. Now raise your hips off the ground while pushing them forward. Now raise your top leg up until your raised leg foot is in line with your top shoulder. This is quite challenging so be sure to maintain a good strong core brace. Now hold this position until you start to shake and feel like you can't keep your core braced and spine supported. If it was less than 20 seconds you should perform 4-5 reps of 20 second planks for 2-3 sets per side. Once you can hold your plank for 30 seconds perform 3-4 reps of 30 second planks for 2-3 sets. Once you can hold your plank for 1 minute or more on both sides do 2-3 sets of 1 minute planks. Once you can achieve a 1 minute plank for 2-3 sets you are strong and stable and ready to move on to more advanced moves such as the Full Side Plank with Lat Rows, Reverse Fly and Dumbbell Reverse Fly.

(A) Full Side Bridge/Plank with Lat Rows

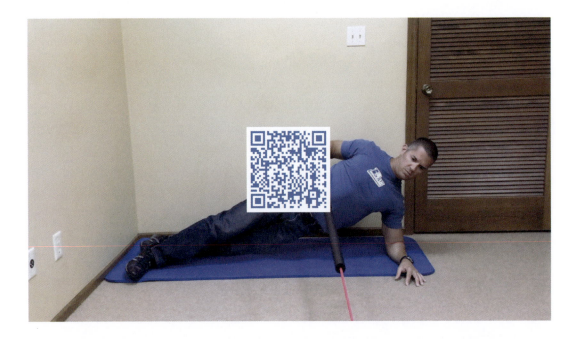

From a side lying position start exactly as per a normal full side bridge/plank. You can use a pully (if you are at a gym or have a home gym) or a band. Brace your core and firmly grab the handle of a connected band or pully with your right hand and simply pull until your hand is at the bottom of your rib cage. There should be no spinal motion or torso twisting. Make sure you set your shoulder blades and keep your neck packed throughout the entire motion. Do 5 reps then switch to your left side. Your goal should be 10-15 reps of lat rows per side for 3 total sets per side.

(A) Full Side Bridge/Plank with Banded Reverse Flys

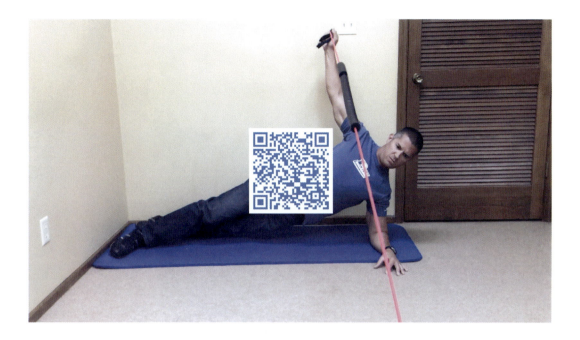

From a side lying position start exactly as per a normal full side bridge/plank. You can use a pully (if you are at a gym or have a home gym) or a band. Brace your core and firmly grab the handle of a connected band or pully with your right hand, now set your shoulder blades, pack your neck and without bending your elbow pull your arm straight up toward the ceiling until your hand is above your shoulder and your arm is straight. There should be no spinal motion or torso twisting. Make sure you set your shoulder blades and keep your neck packed throughout the entire motion. Do 5 reps then switch to your left side. Your goal should be 10-15 reps per side for 3 total sets per side.

(A) Full Side Bridge/Plank with Dumbbell Reverse Flys

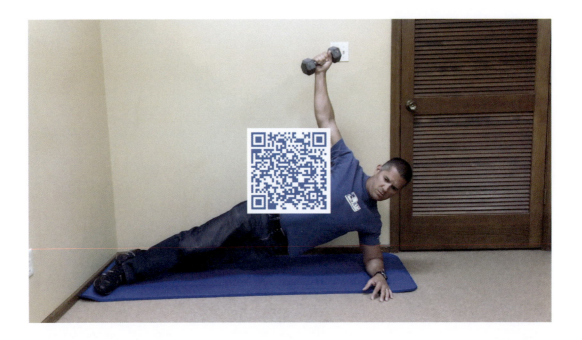

From a side lying position start exactly as per a normal full side bridge/plank. Using a dumbbell that is not too heavy start at the ground with your hand firmly grasping the dumbbell. Now with a strong core brace, shoulder blade set and neck packed raise the dumbbell up with a straight arm until your hand is directly above your shoulder. Hold for a 1 count and without letting go of your stable position slowly lower the dumbbell to the ground. There should be no spinal motion or torso twisting. Make sure you set your shoulder blades and keep your neck packed throughout the entire motion. Do 5 reps then switch to your left side. Your goal should be 10-15 reps per side for 3 total sets per side.

5. Bridge Progressions

(B) Basic Bridge

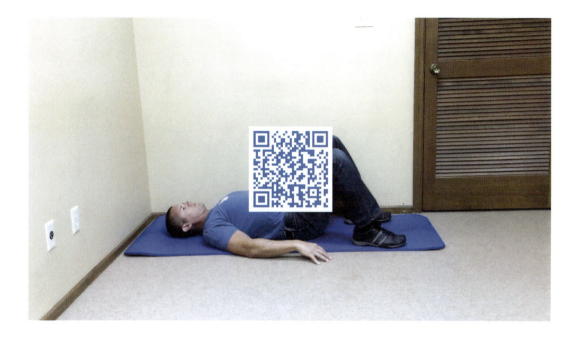

While lying on your back with your feet flat on the floor shoulder width apart and your knees bent allow for a lordotic/curve in your lower back. Now brace your core to ensure no spinal movement takes place during any of the bridge. While maintaining your core brace raise your hips off the ground as you push your knees to the sides about 2-4 inches (this ensures your glutes are doing the work). If you feel as though a hamstring is going to cramp or is cramping go back to the start position and press your knees further out to the side to increase your glute activation. Once there is a straight line from your abs to your quads (thighs) stop and hold this position for 3 seconds. Now without letting go of your core brace lower yourself to the ground. Be sure to not go up too high as you will be potentially hyper extending your spine which may cause some irritation and pain. Your goal should be 12-15 reps for 3 sets with a 3 second hold at the top. Once you can do this you are ready to progress to the Bridge with Leg Extension.

(A) Bridge Single Leg Up Downs

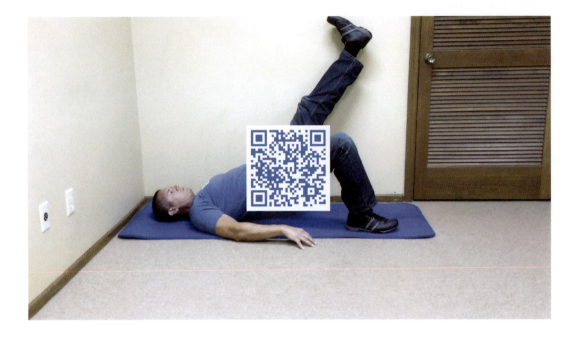

    While lying on your back with your feet flat on the floor shoulder width apart and your knees bent allow for a lordotic/curve in your lower back. Now brace your core to ensure no spinal movement takes place during any of the bridge. While maintaining your core brace, raise your hips off the ground as you push your knees to the sides about 2-4 inches. Now brace your core even harder and push your right foot firmly into the ground as you raise your left leg straight up until your knee is fully extended. You should feel a very strong right glute contraction and an increase in challenge to your core. If your hamstring is cramping on the supported leg you are under-utilizing your glute; simply push your right knee a couple of inches further to the right side and focus on your right glute and you should feel the hamstring relax. Be sure to not go up too high as you will be potentially hyper extending your spine which may cause some irritation and pain. Now with your core brace held, lower your body back to the ground while maintaining the outward position of your knee (to ensure your hamstring doesn't cramp on the way down!). Once you are on the ground, continue to hold your core brace and raise up again on THE SAME SIDE. Perform 10-15 reps per side. Your goal should be 10-15 reps per side for 3 sets.

(A) Bridge From Bench (Hip Thrusters)

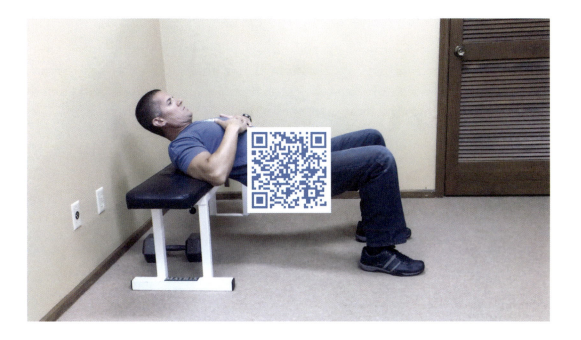

From an exercise bench, couch or bed (please ensure the aforementioned is STABLE AND DOESN'T MOVE) place your shoulder blades and upper back on the object holding you. With your hips bent toward the ground, brace your core, push your knees to the side (to ensure glutes are activating) and raise up until your quads (thighs) and abdominals (stomach) are in a straight line (be sure not to hyper-extend your spine at the top). While maintaining a good core brace hold for 2 seconds and lower yourself back to the start position while pushing your knees to the side. That's 1 rep. Do 10-15 reps with 2 seconds hold at the top for 3 sets.

Standing Core Progressions

Standing core work is just that, exercises that work the core while you are standing/upright. They are slightly more advanced but very practical from the stand point that they teach you to use your core to stabilize while walking, sitting, transitioning and other functions of daily living. As with all of Dr. Rob's "core/back builders" you will need to keep a core brace, shoulder blade/scapular set and neck pack throughout the entire movement.

(I) Suitcase Carry

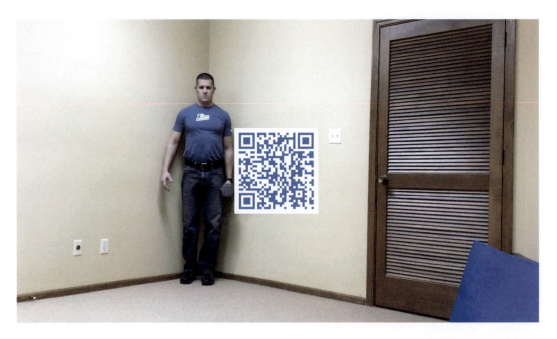

From a standing position pick up a weight, kettle bell or heavy briefcase/bag. The weight should be heavy enough to be challenging but not so heavy that you cannot grip the weight and risk dropping it or you are not keeping good form. As per all of our core moves start with a good core brace, a shoulder blade/scapular set and a packed neck. With your chest raised high simply start walking. You should immediately feel the weight trying to pull you toward its side. As a result your opposite side will contract quite hard to stabilize and protect the spine. Try to walk for 60 seconds. If you feel fatigued prior to 60 seconds or your grip is giving out simply set the weight down (Properly! Mind your back position!) and rest for 10-15 seconds. Time yourself, if you were less than 60 seconds then build up to a goal of 3 sets for 60 seconds each with a weight that is heavy enough to make the last 5-10 seconds quite challenging.

(I) Suitcase Squat

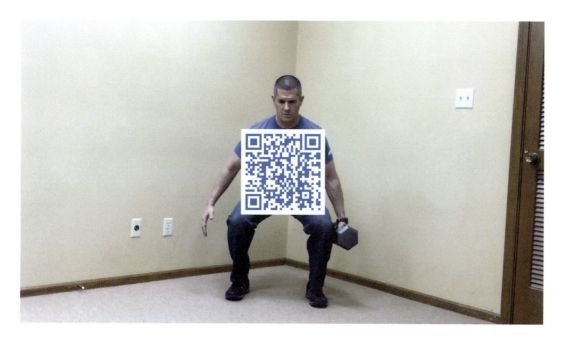

From a standing position pick up a weight, kettle bell or heavy briefcase/bag. The weight should be heavy enough to be challenging but not so heavy that you cannot grip the weight and risk dropping it or you are not keeping good form. As per all of our core moves start with a good core brace, a shoulder blade/scapular set and a packed neck. You can either use a chair/bench/box or nothing at all. From a standing position slowly lower yourself down by pushing your hips and buttocks back as your knees spread apart (be sure to not go too deep or your lower back will round and cause disc issues; if you feel a lower back stretching sensation those are your discs; you've gone too far!). Make sure your knees are not ahead of your toes, if they are push your hips back further. Once you've reached a safe lowered position drive your knees apart and stand up. As with the Suitcase Carry the weight is going to pull you toward its side and your opposite side oblique and QL will have to work really hard to keep you stable. Your goal should be 3 sets of 12-15 reps. Remember form is key here NOT the weight. If you cannot stabilize your core or your form is breaking down, then stop and take a break or lower the weight.

(I) Band Walk out

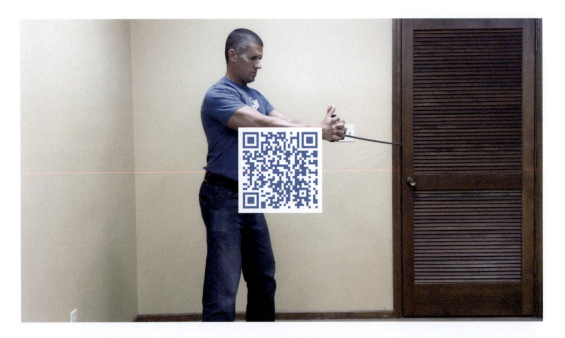

Standing with your left shoulder facing the connection point of a band or pully brace your core, set your scapula and pack your neck and grasp the handle with both hands with fingers interlocked. With your hands just above your navel start to walk sideways away from the connection point until the band feels like it will pull you back to the connection point if you don't remain braced. Now remain braced and stand in an athletic stance with your knees pushing outward (you will feel your glutes contract immediately if this is done properly). While maintaining this position press the handle forward until your arms are straight out in front of you; DON'T LET GO OF YOUR BRACE! Now pull the handle back to your navel and repeat until you are fatigued. Once you are fatigued slowly walk sideways back to the starting point and repeat with your right shoulder facing the connection point. Rest for about 20 seconds (or until you feel recovered) and repeat again on the left side. Your goal should be 12-15 reps of presses per side for 3 sets. Once you can perform this relatively easily try walking out and instead of doing presses with the handle try straightening your arms in front of you (remaining braced!) and do circles, figure 8s, squares and ultimately drawing the alphabet vertically in the air. When you can do 3 sets per side of the full alphabet ranging from your nose to your navel while your arms are straight, you are well on your way to a very strong core and stable spine.

(A) Over-Head Abdominals

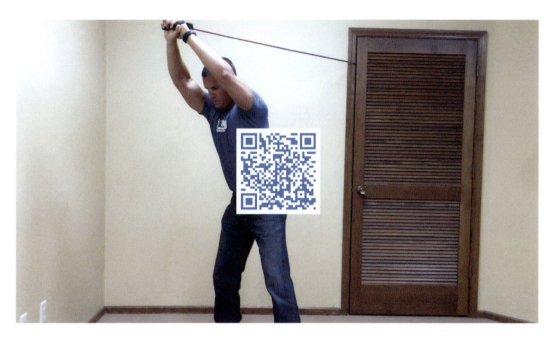

Standing with your back to a band or a pully connection point grasp a handle with both hands so your palms are facing away from you. Walk forward slightly until you feel tension on the band/pully. Brace your core, set your scapula and pack your neck. Raise your arms straight overhead until they are in line with your head. Now slowly push your hips back hinging through your hips until you feel resistance on the band; DON'T GO TOO FAR FOWARD AND LOSE YOUR LOWER BACK

LORDOSIS!! Remain braced and slowly return to the start position. A 6 count back to the start position is ideal for the return. You will feel a big pull on your abdominals going back so make sure you control the movement as this is where the true effect of the exercise is realized. Your goal should be 3 sets of 12-15 reps. Once you can achieve this you are ready for Single Leg Over-Head Abdominals.

(A) Single Leg Over-Head Abdominals

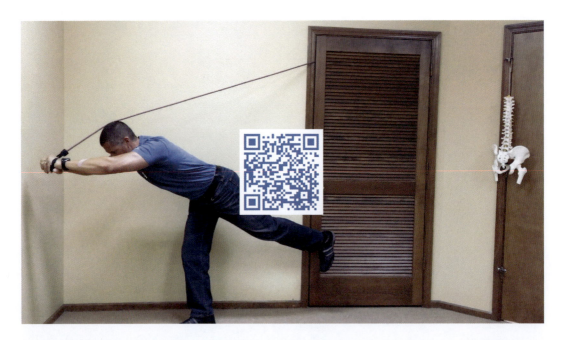

Standing with your back to a band or a pully connection point grasp a handle with both hands so your palms are facing away from you. Walk forward slightly until you feel tension on the band/pully. Brace your core, set your scapula and pack your neck. Raise your arms straight overhead until they are in line with your head. Now balance on your right leg and slowly bend forward through your right hip as your left leg kicks straight back. DON'T GO TOO FAR FOWARD AND LOSE YOUR LOWER BACK LORDOSIS!! Focus on your left glute contracting as it goes back and forward to the start position; this will help with your balance and enable you to stay stable. Return to the start position and finish as many reps as you can while keeping perfect form. Aim for 3 sets of 12-15 reps per leg. If you can accomplish multiple reps and sets of this exercise you not only have a very strong and stable core you have great glute strength and great balance!

Back Breakers

Flexibility Builders

10

Proper Stretching—Knowing How to Recognize Dr. Rob's "Back Breakers" and Dr. Rob's "Flexibility Builders"

SAFE Stretches For Flexibility

So we've corrected your low back problem and you are on the path to feeling better. You've started to train your core safely with Dr. Rob's Core/Back Builders and you are feeling a little tight and want to venture out to a stretching/yoga class at your local gym. STOP!! Please don't attempt a stretching class until you understand how to stretch properly and recognize which stretching poses to avoid. As with core work and activities of daily living stretching should follow the same rules. 1. Move through the hips. 2. Spare the lumbar spine by keeping it in a neutral posture. This means when a yoga instructor tells you to round your spine to touch your toes and come up "vertebra by vertebra" to the upright position you say "NO"! 3. Rotation of the lumbar spine needs to be avoided. If an instructor or a magazine picture has you lay on your back and twist your shoulders one direction and your knees in the other direction, please DON'T! If you follow the list below for a safe and injury free way to stretch, the most common mistakes being made with regard to stretching, you'll be able to achieve a safe and healthy level of flexibility.

Dr. Rob's Back Breaker Stretches

    1. Supine Lumbar Rotation stretch. Places rotational load and strain on the discs and ligaments of the lower back straining them. Even if there is a slight muscle stretch you are causing damage!

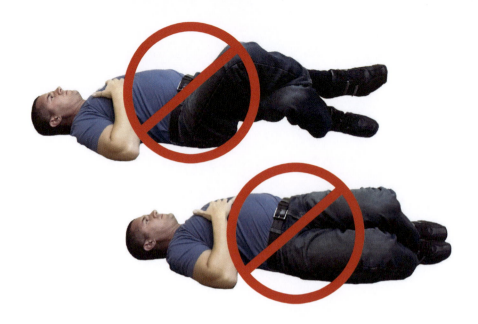

2. Double and Single Knees to Chest. This is still one of the most highly prescribed stretches that I see my patients performing and are often prescribed by other health care practitioners. Again, there is some small muscle stretching but at great risk to the discs and ligaments of already compromised lower backs.

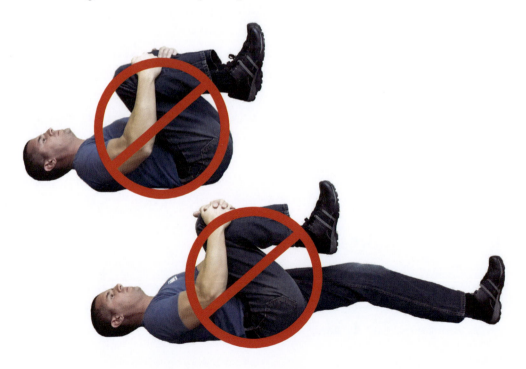

3. I can't state it enough DO NOT BEND OVER TO TOUCH YOUR TOES to stretch your back. I know you were told by your gym teacher in middle school that you should be able to touch your toes! That is complete NONSENSE! IT is NOT functional and it is NOT a measure of fitness! Please use a PROPER hamstring stretch as demonstrated previously to spare your spine.

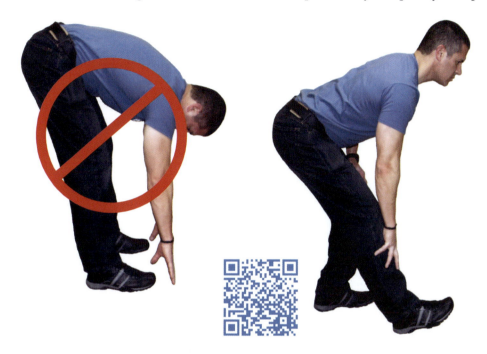

Dr. Rob's Flexibility Builder Stretches

As Stated previously, Dr. Rob's Flexibility Builder Stretches mobilize the areas that are meant to move. As with most stretches a hold of 20-30 seconds per stretch is important to glean the benefit of the stretch. In the following list there are 3 exceptions to the 20-30 second hold rule. The Cat/Camel, Thoracic Chair Extension Mobilization/ Stretch and the Thoracic Rotation Mobilization should be performed with a count of 1,2,3 throughout the movement. For example, while doing the Cat/Camel, think 1,2,3 as you go up and 1,2,3 as you go down. Perform 2-3 reps of 20-30 seconds for the Seated Glute stretches, Psoas stretch, QL/Lat stretch, Hamstring stretch and Standing Quad stretch, and 2-3 sets of 15-20 reps for the Cat/Camel Mobilization stretch, Thoracic Chair Extension Mobilization stretch and Thoracic Rotation stretches.

1. Seated Glute Figure 4 Stretch

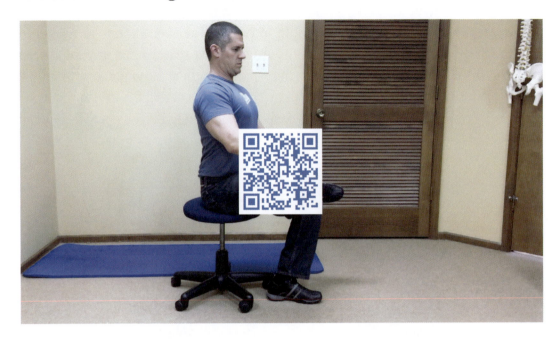

2. Seated Glute Figure 4 Cross Stretch

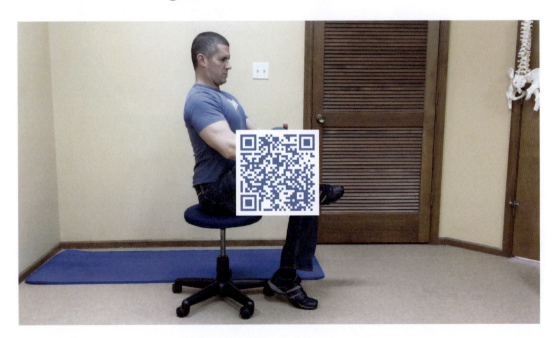

3. Psoas Stretch

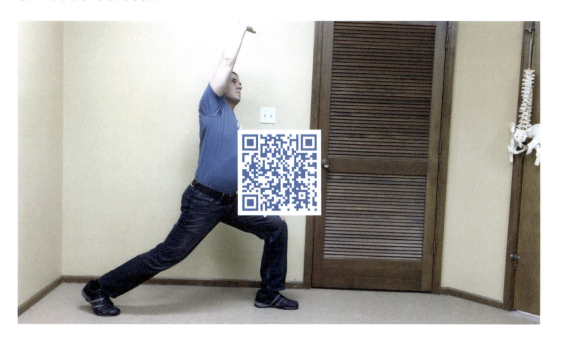

4. QL/Lat Stretch

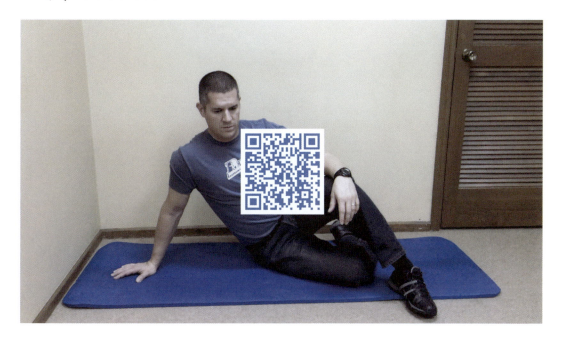

5. Hamstring Stretch

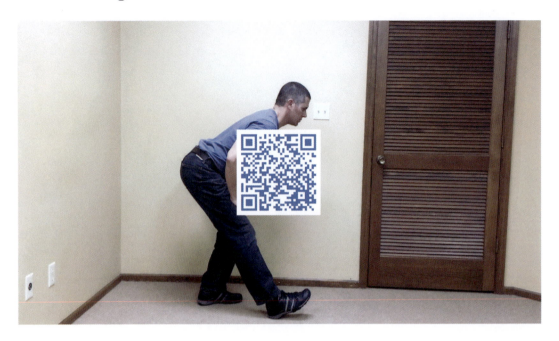

6. Standing Quad Stretch

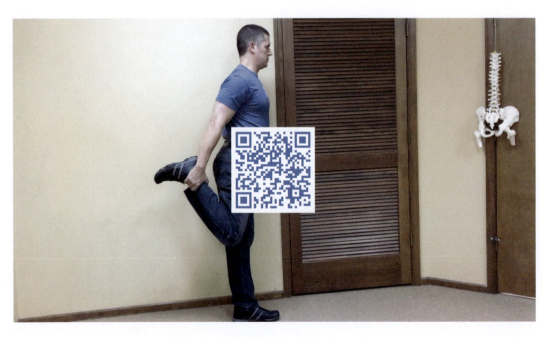

7. Cat/Camel Mobilization Stretch

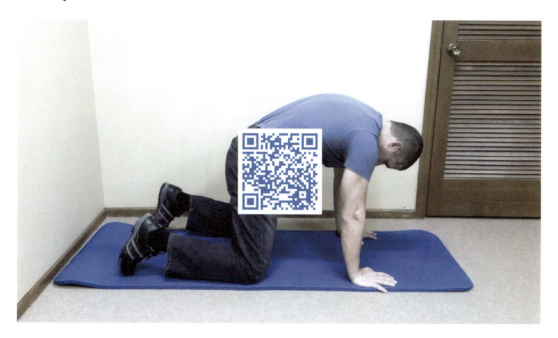

8. Thoracic Chair Extension Mobilization/Stretch

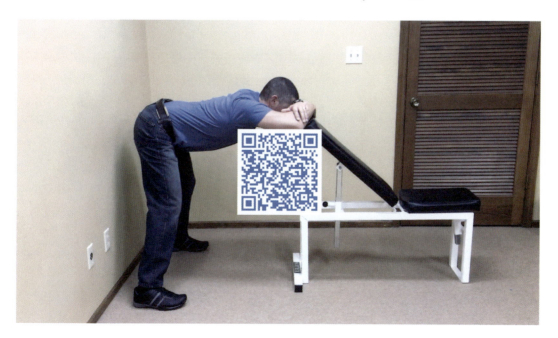

9. Thoracic Rotation Mobilization

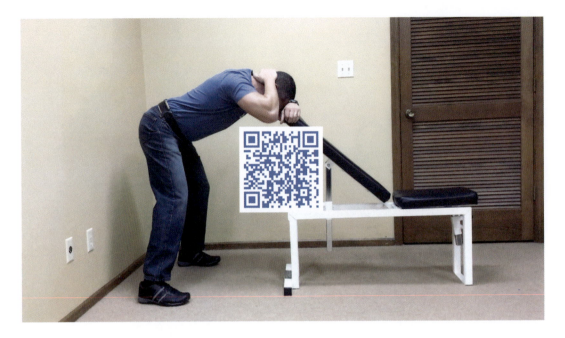

Well here you are, hopefully on your way to feeling less pain in your back and regaining the ability to accomplish physical tasks that may at one time have been arduous at best. If you stick with this plan and learn how to treat your own symptoms, prevent them from coming back with proper daily movement, and build a strong core with safe exercises, you can lift yourself out of the purgatory of being a chronic low back pain sufferer. I'm no different than you are, I've had lower back pain on and off for 25 years. I follow my own advice and the majority of my days are pain free. If I can do it, so can you. I believe in the science, I believe in my program and most of all I believe in you and your body's ability to heal itself, once it is set on the proper path. Good luck and enjoy a healthy back!

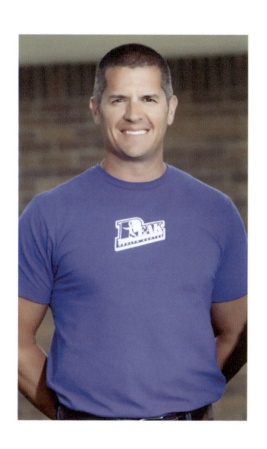

References

Callaghan J and McGill SM. Intervertebral Disc Herniation: Studies on a Porcine Model Exposed To Highly Repetitive Flexion/Extension Motion With Compressive Force. Clinic Bio-Mechanics. 2001; 16 (1): 28-37.

Aultman CD, Scannell J and McGill SM. Predicting the Direction of Nucleus Tracking in Bovine Spine Motion Segments Subjected to Repetitive Flexion and Simultaneous Lateral Bend. Clinical Bio-Mechanics. 2005; 20: 126-129.

Cholewick, J, Lulum K and McGill SM. The Intra-Abdominal Pressure Mechanism For Stabilizing the Lumbar Spine. Journal of Bio-Mechanics. 1999; 32 (1): 13-17.

Valouchova PT, Liebenson C. Self-Management: Patient Section the New Abdominals. Journal of Body Work and Movement Therapies. 2009; 13: 112-113.

Marras WS, Parrianpour M, Ferguson SA et al. The Classification of Anatomic and Symptomatic Based Low-Back Disorders Using Motion Measure Models. Spine. 1995; 20: 2531-2546.

Wetzel FT, Donelson R. The Role of Repeated End Range Pain Response Assessment in the Management of Symptomatic Lumbar Discs. The Spine Journal. 2003; 3: 146-154.

Mooney V, Dressinger TE. Evidence-Informed Management of Chronic Low Back Pain with Lumbar Strengthening and Mckenzie Exercises. Critical Reviews in Physical Rehabilitation. 2008; 20 (4): 323-341.

Grenier SG, McGill SM. Quantification of Lumbar Stability By Using Two Different Abdominal Strategies. Archives in Physical Medicine. 2007; 88 (1): 54-62.

Beattie PF, Arnot CF, Dooley JW, Noda H, Baily L. The Immediate Reduction in Low Back Pain Intensity Following Lumbar Joint Mobilization and Prone Press-ups is Associated With Increased Diffusion of Water in the L5-S1 Disc. Journal of Orthopedics and Sports Physical Therapy. 2010; 40 (5): 256-264.

Watanabe S, Eguchi A, Kobura K, Ishida H. Influence of Trunk Muscle Co-Contraction On Spinal Curvature During Sitting For Desk Work. Electromyographic Clinical Neurophysiology. 2007; 47 (6): 273-278.

Lee SU, Fredericson M, Butts K, Lang P. The Effect of Axial Loading and Spine Position on Intervertebral Disc Hydration: An in Vivo Pilot Study. Journal of Back and Muskuloskeletal Rehabilitation. 2005; 18: 15-20.

Adams MA, May S, Freeman BJ. Effects of Backward Bending on Lumbar Intervertebral Discs: Relevance to Physical Therapy Treatments for Low Back Pain. Spine. 2010; 25 (4): 431-438.

Sengal N, Fortin JD. Internal Disc Disruption and Low Back Pain. Pain Physician. 2000; 3 (2): 143-157.

Donelson R. The Mckenzie Approach to Evaluating and Treating Low Back Pain. Orthopedic Review. 1990; 19: 681-686.

Scannell JP and McGill SM. Disc Prolapse. Evidence of Reversal With Repeated Extensions. Spine. 2009; 34 (4): 344-350.

Morningstar MW. Strength Gains Through Lumbar Lordosis Restoration. Journal of Chiropractic Medicine. 2003; 2 (4): 137-141.

Cholewicki J, Julunu K, Mcgill SM. The Intra-Abdominal Pressure Mechanism For Stabilizing The Lumbar Spine. Journal of Biomechanics. 1999; 32(1): 13-17.

Roma SM, Nagrale S, Dabadghen R. Assessment of Lumbar Lordosis and Lumbar Core Strength in Information Technology Professionals. Asian Spine Journal. 2016; 10 (3): 495-500.

MiyazakiJ, Marata S, Horie J et al. Lumbar Lordosis Angle and Leg Strength Predict Walking Ability in Elderly Males. Archives in Gerontology and Geriatrics. 2013; 56 (1): 141-147.

McGill, Stuart. Low Back Disorders. Evidence Based Prevention and Rehabilitation. Human Kinetics. 2007.

Cholewicki J and McGill SM. Lumbar Posterior Ligament Involvement During Extremely Heavy Lifts Estimated From Fluoroscopic Measurements. Journal of Biomechanics. 1999; 25 (1): 17-28.

Reed CA, Ford KR, Myer GD et al. The Effects of Isolated and Integrated Core Stability Training on Athletic Performance Measures: A systematic Review. Sports Medicine. 2012; 42 (8): 697-706.

Abdelrouf OR, Abdel-Aziem AA. The Relationship Between Core Endurance and Back Dysfunction in Collegiate Male Athletes With and Without Non-specific Low Back Pain. International Journal of Sports Therapy. 2016; 11 (3): 337-344.

Department of Public and Occupational Health and Institute for Health and Care Research, VU University Medical Center, Amsterdam, The Netherlands. Back Pain: Prevention and Management in the Workplace. Best Practices in Clinical Rheumatology. 2015; 29 (3): 483-494.

Allread WG, Waters TR. Interventions to Reduce Low-Back Injury Risk Among Youth Who Perform Feed Handling and Scooping Tasks on Farms. Journal of Agricultural Safety and Health. 2007; 13 (4): 375-393.

Calatayard J, Casara J et al. Trunk Muscle Activity During Different Variations of the Supine Plank Exercise. Muskuloskeletal Scientific Practice. 2017; (28): 54-58.

Hides JA, Jull GA, Richardson CA. Long-Term Effect of Specific Stabilizing Exercises for First Episode Low-Back Pain. Spine. 2016; 26: 243-248.

Coulombe BJ, Games KE, Neil ER, Eberman LE. Core Stability Exercises Versus General Exercise For Chronic Low Back Pain. Journal of Athletic Training. 2017; 52 (1): 71-71.

Liebenson Craig. Rehabilitation of the Spine. Lippincott, Williams and Wilkens. 2007.

Key J, Cliff A, Cordie F, Hauley C. A Model of Movement Dysfunction Provides a Classification System Guiding Diagnosis and Therapeutic Care in Spinal Pain and Related Musculoskeletal Syndromes. Journal of Body Work and Movement Therapy. 2008; 12 (1): 7-21.

Youdas, JW, Buor MM et al. Surface Electromyographic Analysis of Core Trunk and Hip Muscles During Selected Rehabilitation Exercises in the Side-Bridge to Neutral Position. Sports Health. 2014; 6 (5): 416-421.

Ekstrom RA, Donatelli RA, CAP KC. Electromyographic Analysis of Core Trunk Hip and Thigh Muscles During 9 Rehabilitation Exercises. Journal of Orthopedic Sports Physical Therapy. 2007; 37 912): 754-762.

Boren K, Courney C, LeCoquic J et al. Electromyographic Analysis of Gluteus Medius and Gluteus Maximus During Rehabilitation Exercises. International Journal of Sports Physical Therapy. 2011; 6 (3): 206-223.

Distefano LJ, Blackburn JT, Contreras B. Gluteal Muscle Activation During Common Therapeutic Exercises. Journal of Orthopedic Sports Physical Therapy. 2009; 39 (7): 532-540.

Macadam P, Cronin J, Contreras b. An Examination of the Gluteal Muscle Activity Associated With Dynamic Hip Abduction and Hip External Rotation Exercise: A Systematic Review. International Journal of Sports Physical Therapy. 2015; 10 (5): 573-591.

Theodoidis T, Kramer J, Kleinert H. Conservative Treatment of Lumbar Spine Stenosis. A Review. Orthopedics. 2008; 146 (1): 75-79.

Ammendola C, Chow N. Clinical Outcomes For Neurogenic Claudication Using A Multi-Modal Program for Lumbar Spinal Stenosis. Journal of Manipulative and Physiologic Therapeutics. 2015; 38: 188-194.

Axler C and McGill SM. Low Back Loads Over a Variety of Abdominal Exercises: Searching for the Safest Abdominal Challenge. Medicine and Science in Sports and Exercise. 1997; 29 (6): 804-811.

(Waterloo's Dr. Spine, Stuart McGill). (2011, October 27). Retrieved from http://www.youtube.com/watch?v=0330gPH6NNE.

(Gray Cook: Motor Control, Stability and Prime Mover Training). (2013, October 16). Retrieved from https://www.youtube.com/watch?v=xf9CD214fIK.

Printed in Poland
by Amazon Fulfillment
Poland Sp. z o.o., Wrocław

22843448R00098